12 Pa Myths:

Eat Better than a Caveman

A proud presentation of:

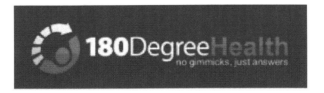

April 2013
Copyright © 2013 180DegreeHealth, LLC. All rights reserved worldwide.
ISBN 1490571507
ISBN-13: 978-1490571508

DISCLAIMER

The material provided here is for educational and informational purposes only and is not intended as medical advice. The information contained in this eBook should not be used to diagnose or treat any illness, metabolic disorder, disease, or health problem. If you have developed a serious illness of some kind, the complexities of dealing with that disorder are best handled by your physician or other professional health care provider, whom you should also consult with before beginning any nutrition or exercise program. Use of the programs, advice, and other information contained in this eBook is at the sole choice and risk of the reader.

4

Contents

Introduction	7
Paleo – The Typical Physiological Scenario	13
You! On Paleo!	21
Intermittent Fasting	25
Signs and Symptoms of Paleo Gone Wrong	30
12 Paleo Myths	51
A Natural Diet is Superior	53
We are Genetically Identical to How We Were 100,000 Years Ago	60
Agriculture Made Us Small and Weak	68
Carbs Cause "Insidious Weight Gain"	73
Insulin Resistant People Store More Glycogen	81

Hunter Gatherers Had Sexy Bodies	91
Carbohydrates Cause Insulin Resistance	105
Low-carb Diets Ensure Low Glucose and Insulin Levels	113
Lack of Genetic Adaptation to Modern Foods Causes Food Sensitivities	121
Burning Fat as Fuel is Superior	130
High Protein Diets Raise Your Metabolism	134
It is Healthy to Lose Weight on a Paleo Diet	138
A Quick Primer on How to Overcome Paleo-itis	148
Paleo Fails	153
Other Books and Audio Programs by Matt Stone	223
References	224

Introduction

Now now, take it easy caveman/woman. I know I have a tendency to drive you Paleophiles up the wall, but hear me out. What you are about to read is simply a tale of reality, not the typical science fiction (more like science out of context) that dominates the fields of health and nutrition in popular books and websites.

For those of you who aren't already clued in to what the concept driving the popular "Paleo diet" is, here's a quick primer...The Paleo Diet is a broad term that encompasses eating pretty much anything other than grains and dairy products and modern, processed foods – from Cheetos to Mountain Dew and everything in between.

The basic premise that fuels this concept, which also has an exercise and lifestyle component that typically accompanies it in an attempt to mimic what daily life was probably like during the Paleolithic era, is quite simple. The belief is that humans genetically evolved during this roughly 2.5 million year period, and our DNA or genetic "blueprint," was created during this time. Then came the end of the Paleolithic era and a massive amount of changes that our genes simply haven't been able to keep up with. In terms of food, this includes many major agricultural products (milk, cheese, other milk-based products, corn, wheat, soy, rice, oats, and so on) with an even more stringent avoidance of the super-modern processed, packaged, and flavor-enhanced foods manufactured by the food industry. You also see the recommendation to avoid nightshade vegetables and legumes due to phytochemicals (plant poisons) contained therein considered to be harmful and inflammation-causing.

Thus, the basic staples of the Paleo Diet are things that can be hunted and gathered. A little leafy matter is good. Meat and fish – excellent, especially meat from animals that live and eat similar to their natural diet and lifestyle. Nuts and seeds are an easy thing to gather certain times of year and are championed. And finally, fruit and berries. This grows on trees and bushes at various times of the year and can easily be picked and eaten without any preparation – it doesn't get much more Paleo than this.

Sure, this is the basic backbone. And this is basically the premise of one of the first major books written by a Colorado State University professor named Loren Cordain. The title of the book – The Paleo Diet of course. Way to keep it simple doc!

But the details are of course relentlessly masturdebated by the Paleo community. Some negative scientific data comes out on say, fructose, and then the Paleo community scrambles to come up with explanations. A couple of common explanations that were served up to explain this were:

1) Fruits during that era were not hybridized for such massive sweetness like modern fruits in supermarkets today
2) Paleo man only ate fruits seasonally, and not 365 days per year

And of course others claim that studies, particularly those involving rodents and totally unnatural amounts of fructose in highly-refined form, are not relevant and cannot be equated to fructose found with an abundance of fiber and nutrition found in natural fruits and berries. I'm sure little squabbles like this will abound for decades before this modern diet craze starts to fizzle into obscurity. But this kind of describes the sort of limbo that the diet resides in – one where scientific discovery is constantly being passed through a sort of Paleolithic litmus test, and the thing just keeps getting more muddled and confused – the lines graying more and more as Paleo keeps chugging along and stopping to pick up new passengers.

Since they sort of make up the rules as they go along, Paleo could really be used to endorse just about anything. New discoveries come out and the Paleo community tries to own it by saying "Paleo man musta done that! It's in our DNA to fast intermittently!" Likewise, any criticisms that anyone might have can be easily deflected. My criticisms of Paleo are immediately met with lines like, "Paleo doesn't mean low-carb," or "you don't have to fast for it to be Paleo." Pretty soon eating ice cream will be Paleo. Oh wait, Robb Wolf and Mark Sisson, the two biggest Paleo celebs, have already posted a picture of the two of them eating ice cream together.

So, Paleo is one thing in premise. In reality it is something that could be just about anything.

Anyway, that's the basics of what the Paleo diet and lifestyle is. This book is about challenging some of the components of the Paleo diet that are:

- Scientifically inaccurate – such as the belief that carbohydrates raise blood sugar and insulin levels

- Built on assumption – such as the belief that the typical human diet from 100,000 years ago MUST be the optimal diet
- Built on a false premise – such as the belief that if every society eats grains and has inflammatory diseases, then grains must be the cause of those inflammatory diseases
- And so on

What this book is, is far less important than WHY I decided to write it. I decided to write this book specifically because of the increasing popularity and positivity surrounding the Paleo diet and lifestyle. I am fully aware that a diet that removes either grains, dairy products, nightshade vegetables, legumes, or a combination can be therapeutic for certain health problems – certainly in the short-term when it comes to eliminating symptoms. I am also fully aware that many experience substantial and undeniable improvements, particularly in the first 6-12 months of eating a diet based more on meat and vegetables and less on grains and sugars. I am also aware of the benefits many experience from switching from a junk food-based diet, low in nutrients and high in industrial chemicals, oxidized fats, and other nasties to a very nutritious, whole foods diet. Paleo gives them a compelling intellectual reason to try, and to stick with, the diet. It's a fun group, with a great community feel – leaving its followers feeling "in the know" and empowered over the rest of the mortals eating and living "normal."

Note – I acknowledge, fully, that in some cases a Paleo diet may very well be the IDEAL nutritional, scratch that, MEDICAL intervention for some people and their health problems. Its rise in popularity is something that we should all be thankful for. It has provided solutions to many in need and unable to find it until it rose out of obscurity and more into the public eye. This book is not about negating, downplaying, overlooking, or attempting to "take down" the Paleo movement.

This book, to be crystal clear, is written to bring attention to some of the negatives of the diet - to highlight the risks and dangers that are either covered up, ignored, or just plain not understood by the top public figures in the Paleosphere. It is written as a slap in the face for those who have convinced themselves Paleo is the way, but are ignoring overt signs that their health is being adversely affected by it – especially with prolonged adherence. It is written as a lifeline for those who are not getting answers from the Paleo community about why they are experiencing health problems, or why their health problems are not going away, by following the Paleo commandments.

I have communicated with many people, particularly young people, who had their health, social life, and sanity completely decimated by entering into the Paleo world. I have answered thousands of emails and have communicated with people of all ages and genders all over the globe in the 50,000 comments on my site. Failure on a Paleo diet, particularly when carbohydrates are restricted as is so often the case with the generally negative bias against them in the Paleo community, is not uncommon. It is VERY common, and the reasons for it are a matter of simple human physiology.

As my understanding of how the human body works has evolved in my own extensive health exploration, I have also become particularly adept at helping those that developed problems on a Paleo diet to overcome those problems – and overcome them very quickly and efficiently. It's not exactly rocket science. It's very simple actually – in most cases.

Before we get into a dozen "Paleo Myths" that I have selected for the purpose of helping you to start peeling back the layers of your tunnel vision regarding the seeming infallibility of Paleo logic, I would like to start this badboy with a very simple breakdown of the physiological reasons why you or someone else you know, is having problems on a Paleo regime. I will of course go over the many different signs that emerge first when Paleo starts to crossover into Faileo territory, and what these signs symbolize from a broader physiological perspective.

I have included lots of personal accounts of Paleo failures from emails and comments I've received as well, just to help you see that some of these things I talk about are not make believe, but happen regularly, and, more importantly – predictably.

And, if you're lucky, I will highlight at the end some quick tips on how to recover from some of the problems incurred on a Paleo diet. This will scare the hell out of you, because the top priority is getting out of a high stress, sympathetic dominant state as quickly as possible. And health food sucks at helping you do that! So does exercise. Part of it is to overcome the infatuation with natural foods and phobias you have about modern foods as well, which I guarantee has become terribly imbalanced since you began on your primal quest. I will just tell it like it is, and, due to your lack of experience with recovering from metabolic issues, you will probably disagree. I would love for us to agree, but then we'd both be wrong! I of course have many other materials on the how's and why's of metabolic recovery if you find that section unconvincing enough to actually saddle up to a pizza and root beer float.

Anyway, hop in the Delorean Marty McFly, and let's go back to the future.

Paleo – The Typical Physiological Scenario

This chapter may give you a headache. It is pretty simple, but it may not seem that way. The short answer is that Paleo tends to increase adrenal activity (increased glucocorticoid production as well as catecholamines – like epinephrine, norepinephrine, and dopamine – the same chemicals released when taking amphetamines/stimulants or during stress), due to increased consumption of animal protein and fat and decreased consumption of carbohydrates – and because a whole foods diet spontaneously decreases calorie consumption (and absorption) for most people – putting their bodies into a catabolic state (high adrenal state).

The common practices of intermittent fasting and exercise magnifies this effect. This leads to some very powerful and noticeable physiological, mental, and emotional changes – from effortless weight loss and a decrease in inflammation to incredible mood and energy enhancement. At least for a while (the "catecholamine honeymoon" I call it), usually about 6 months, but this honeymoon period can fail to be triggered completely in those with weak adrenal glands, or it can go on for quite some time in those with energizer bunny adrenals.

Nothing is 100% set in stone either. It's not like everyone experiences an increase in catecholamines on a Paleo diet. If it is high enough in calories and carbs, it might be fine. Others with impaired glucose metabolism who are used to having big stress hormone surges throughout the day during hypoglycemic episodes, see a decrease in adrenal activity and maybe even a drop in glucocorticoid production (don't get too shortsighted on me here though – just because one can "control" erratic blood sugar on a high-protein diet doesn't make this the optimal solution – which would be to fix the impaired glucose metabolism). A Paleo diet might even stop catabolism (breaking down), and trigger impressive, spontaneous growth of muscle tissue and bone in such a scenario. So it does depend, to some extent, on context and the individual in which the Paleo diet is interacting with.

Individual differences aside, here's an attempt to sort of simplify how things play out in a typical case of someone who needs to drop Paleo like a bad habit. As you will see, the amazing short-term improvements make Paleo incredibly alluring, and are what keep many people frustratingly tinkering around with various permutations of the Paleo diet – often going lower and lower in carbs, until he or she is totally metabolically fucked (TMF). Please excuse the complex medical terminology[1].

---

[1] Don't worry, to keep from offending anyone I have decided not to use Tim Tebow's name in vain at any point in this manuscript, or use the word "chink" when talking about anything that might have something to do with the New York Knicks. Or say anything derogatory about bitches, ho's, retards, midgets, cripples, or Richard Nikoley's mom.

Before we start, let's examine my own personal experience with eating a diet that shared many commonalities with a typical Paleo diet and lifestyle…

Me and My Good Paleo

In 2007 I began researching and writing about the virtues of ancestral diets, animal products, and diets in which fat contributed to a larger percentage of dietary calories ingested – in the meantime becoming increasingly down on modern food processing and many commercial agricultural staples. Although I wasn't completely dairy and grain-free during this time, my intake of such foods aside from butter and an occasional slice or two of sprouted bread was very minimal. My typical carbohydrate intake was about 100-150 grams per day – smack in the middle of Mark Sisson's optimal carbohydrate safe zone. My food quality was second to none. I obtained almost everything I ate from local farms – grassfed and pastured everything. Even some biodynamics in there. One summer I managed to go 3 months without even buying anything at a grocery store except a jar of coconut oil. Everything came exclusively from local farms and farmer's markets.

In a matter of days I was waking up at dawn with tons of energy for the first time in my life. My skin got crystal clear. My teeth started feeling strong, with less pain and sensitivity – and they got whiter – even though I wasn't brushing my teeth every day like I had my entire life prior to that point. I had always had a major sugar addiction, or so it felt like. I could never have sugary foods in the house without plowing through them all until they were gone in a frenzy – regardless of the quantity. At one point I had even gone through a phase of eating handfuls of Halloween candy every day with an entire chocolate bar – so much chocolate in fact, that I had to start ordering it in bulk!

But the most amazing thing happened. I opened up my cabinets on the 4th day and saw two chocolate bars sitting on the shelves that I had completely forgotten about. I took a few bites and lost interest. I found them once again several weeks later, with the opened bar looking white and crumbly from having gotten somewhat stale. This was the first time this had ever happened in my life. I was totally free, from the beginning, from hunger, cravings, desires for alcohol, stimulants, or sweets, etc. It was a totally mind-blowing experience.

In the first couple of months, my mood was incredible. I had always had a very dynamic mood, swinging from great highs to great lows – especially after my first "healthy" eating endeavors with Donna Gates's *Body Ecology Diet* and a series of "cleanses" inspired primarily by Kevin Trudeau – leaving me weak, undermuscled, and depleted with harder to manage mood fluctuations. Working many years as a Wilderness Ranger was no help either – as each grueling season seemed to strip off a small layer of muscle, particularly in the upper body, and replace it with a small extra layer of cushion.

But this new dietary change eliminated that completely. No more roller coaster ride. Just rock solid – even keel and focused. It seemed nothing could throw that off course. It was fantastic.

And then there was my body. I wasn't doing this for any improvement in body composition. I mean, if I was looking to gain some muscle I probably would have been lifting weights – doing more than an occasional round of pushups and situps, going on walks, and snorkeling. But I wasn't. Yet, my shirts (t-shirts mostly, my wardrobe is on par with Beavis and Butthead's) kept getting tighter and tighter, especially in the chest, shoulders, and sleeves. My pants and shorts were practically sliding off of me though, and I was not dating anyone at the time, so it had to have been what I was eating.

What else? My asthma improved. Crazy erections in the beginning that kept me awake at night sometimes. I had no gas, bloating, or stomach pain for the first time in my life. I think I farted about 3 times in the first 6 months. Flawless. I did work another season as a Wilderness Ranger too, and I lost no muscle mass for the first time ever, but became stupidly ripped, with a full 6-pack without doing a single situp.
It was, in short, insane. It was like being on steroids because I WAS on steroids. My own. I have no doubts that I saw a substantial increase in testosterone, growth hormone, DHEA, and all that good stuff in the beginning. This was, without question, a big improvement from the predominantly vegetarian diet I had eaten in the past, interspersed with vegan "cleanses" to make sure I was extra starving. This is a common theme too, as many who report doing wonderfully on a Paleo diet, with instant and dramatic results similar to mine, are those coming from a painful rice, bean, and soy past – like Robb Wolf. Paleo is a powerful antidote for a poorly-designed vegetarian diet, especially one like mine that I combined with 50 hours of "cardio" per week.

In fact, I would say that my response to a diet and lifestyle that was, for all practical purposes, pretty much indistinguishable from say, Mark Sisson's *Primal Blueprint*, was as good as anyone's that I have known or read about. How good? Good enough to rush to write a book and start a website business selling it in a mad dash to save the peoples of the earth of all their health problems.

But 4-5 months in, early signs of failure started to creep in. Boners went from pure steel to sort of mediocre half-empty tubes of toothpaste. My teeth started hurting. I got some zits on my back. Awaking at dawn with energy changed to waking at 4am feeling wired, with dark circles forming under my eyes. There were a few irrational temper tantrums having nothing to do with anything circumstantial – like the old days but worse. Sugar cravings started coming back – unfortunate as anything sweet caused my forehead to become littered with pimples unlike when I consumed sweets prior to embarking on this magical new perfect diet. Speaking of sweets, even a single banana would cause extreme emotional swings and crying fits – not too becoming of a 29-year old stallion.

And dear Lord was the body odor, breath odor, and indigestion relentless. Even a single sip of water 3 hours after a meal would give me a sudden surge of acid in my throat. I felt like I had to sweat 2 quarts a day to flush out the nasty smell that radiated from my pits. The taste in my mouth was rough, and the girl that fell hopelessly for a Manimal of *Fight Club*-caliber awesomeness during the honeymoon period was now requesting that I brush my teeth every 5 minutes, and date someone else while I'm at it.

Let's see what else? Asthma came back. I got puffy for a while, gaining back some weight and watching my abs disappear and my eyes get all puffy and swollen. All kinds of good stuff.

Hey, no worries though. It obviously wasn't working so I just ditched it and tried something else. Errr, not so much. I gave it another 2 full years, hoping that I might accidentally start feeling just like I did at the beginning. But it kept on getting worse, at least when I tried hard. And when it comes to a Paleo type of diet and trying hard, that usually means upping the fat and protein even more and going even lower in carbs. You know, getting really strict about avoiding those grains and sugars and milk. In December of 2008, I went Zero Carb for a whole month.

Interestingly, when I had an occasional binge on juice or candy bars or went out for a few beers I felt great, for a day or two.

It wasn't until I visited my brother for a few days and refused to let my diet interfere with us hanging out and doing our bro thing, that I really started having to face reality. At the time my brother ate a lot of fast food. I watched him dip a cookie into a glass of Blue Powerade once. I just said screw it for those few days and ate like him. My asthma improved. Heartburn improved. Mood improved. Skin got clearer. Slept better. Trust me, being a health researcher and advocate of farm-fresh organic food, having health problems incurred on what you think is the perfect diet clear up eating at Krystal and McDonald's is like being bludgeoned in the taint with a Garden Weasel. But I still didn't come around on something as simple as "carbs" for quite a while – not until 2009 when caution was fully thrown to the wind regarding macronutrients and I started eating plenty of "everything," only to find a severe indigestion problem of 4 years clearing up in 72 hours… among many other benefits.

Anyway, what the hell happened? How could I go from superhero to total mess eating a very nutritious, whole foods, fresh-from-the farm diet? How can you see health improvements on a diet and then ruin your health eating the exact same way? How can a junk food diet give you mediocre health all your life and then, later, actually improve your health? Why did my teeth undergo great improvements on a zero refined sugar diet, then hurt like hell on a zero refined sugar diet, and then later improve dramatically by adding refined sugar to my diet? I mean, preventing tooth demineralization by adding white sugar to your diet? That's insane!

But it is reality. It is what happened to me. And what really happened to me is a lot more meaningful to me personally than what any logic or study may have revealed. It doesn't take a study to convince me that it hurts to get punched in the face. Likewise, a study that showed me that getting punched in the face doesn't hurt, and that during the Paleolithic era humans evolved to feel no pain when punched in the face, wouldn't mean a damn thing to me – especially with 50,000 comments on my blog of other people noticing that it does, indeed, hurt to get punched in the face. So, without further ado, let us look next at what many years of searching and racking my brain about the physiological mechanisms behind what I and so many others have experienced with this type of dietary change – both short-term and long-term, has yielded…

You! On Paleo!

My best description of what happens, in a typical Paleo crash case, goes something like this…

There are hundreds of ways to increase your production of catecholamines. Catecholamines make you feel absolutely awesome. Doing methamphetamine, for example, raises catecholamines through the roof. They feel so good that you are likely to become so addicted to the feeling that you will ruin your life in pursuit of it.

Catecholamines blunt appetite while increasing fat mobilization (fat burning). The best supplement ever created to achieve this was Ephedra, an herbal amphetamine. It worked pretty well for a lot of people. I once worked in the supplement industry[2] after Ephedra was banned. I must have heard 300 people bitch about how Ephedra was removed from the market. Not only did it help people to lose weight without hunger, and have legendary workouts, it made people feel superhuman – with great mental focus and energy.

This should sound familiar to those who started out great on the Paleo diet, or any diet that restricts carbohydrates or

---

[2] I was young! I needed the money!

calories – even slightly. Note, this is not the only way to achieve this. You can achieve this effect on Weight Watchers too, or through hard exercise, or through fasting, stimulant use, stress, or an uber low-fat diet. Eating disorders with super low calorie intakes are notorious for triggering this surge of catecholamines. Because of the addiction that develops, it becomes very difficult to resume eating food – as this triggers withdrawal symptoms with a big crash in mood and accompanying sluggishness, brain fog, and other negatives to accompany the digestive pains, bloating, and reactive hypoglycemia. This is the primary reason why eating disorders are self-perpetuating. But that's a whole other topic.

Anyway, the Paleo diet, with its negative attitude about carbohydrates and insulin, often results in a meat and vegetable-based diet amongst its followers. Protein stimulates more of the stress response of the human body, including releasing glucagon – a blood sugar increasing hormone that is part of the overall stress response. You also see some gluconeogenesis occurring, converting protein and muscle tissue into glucose for use in the brain, and some in the muscles. This effect is magnified when carbohydrates are not present. Carbohydrates tend to "spare" protein, allowing it to enter into muscle cells as amino acids. Consuming protein by itself causes a portion to get broken down into glucose, which I believe becomes more and more prevalent the more the body gets to "practice" making this conversion. I make this point because at first the body isn't good at breaking down your muscle tissue for glucose, but the more practice it gets the more it starts breaking down muscle tissue over time – thus, at first you may maintain or even build muscle but this can reverse itself eventually.

In short, high calorie intakes with lots of carbs stimulate insulin production – a powerful pro-thyroid, pro-metabolic hormone that puts us into a parasympathetic-dominant state, where growth occurs, carbohydrate storage occurs, and youthful anabolic hormones rise (like DHEA, testosterone, etc.), and the adrenals relax. Think of how sleepy and relaxed and warm and cozy you feel after Thanksgiving feast. That's the anti-stress, pro-thyroid, growth state of the body. A male after orgasm should be entering this state, and feeling these feelings as well (warmth, relaxation, thousand-pound eyelids).

A meal with lots of protein and very little carbohydrate does the opposite – leaving us feeling alert, energized, with fat burning up and catabolic hormones active. Those are virtues promoted by advocates of a low-carb diet, but this pro-stress hormone state has a lot of unwanted negative side effects, the least of which is accelerated aging, the worst of which is atrophy of the thymus and thyroid, demineralization of teeth and bone, impaired immune system (increased development of allergy and autoimmunity), decrease in sex hormones, DHEA, and other known youth hormones, and a host of other negatives. Basically the same side effects as abuse of stimulants. And this is just all part of the stress response of the body, what many scientists, such as Hans Selye, Ray Peat, or Robert Sapolsky would agree is the root cause of most common illnesses.

You eventually become desensitized to these hormones and neurotransmitters or stop producing so much of them (adrenal fatigue/burnout/Addison's disease) or both. In fact, to highlight this effect, in a discussion of the most exhaustive studies ever done on calorie restriction, the author (Ancel Keys) mentions that starving men injected with adrenaline noticed no effect from it! This is why the more stimulants you take in the more you need to continue taking in to get a rise from it…

"In 40 persons who received subcutaneous injections of 1 mg. of adrenalin there was extraordinarily little response to the drug."

Note, these men didn't achieve this effect by taking stimulants per se, but via exposure to high amounts of catecholamines through weight loss induced by a calorie level that, by the way, is higher than what most weight loss "experts" recommend (about 1,600 per day).

Along similar lines, the longer you do "Paleo" the more the honeymoon effect that you noticed initially starts to fade, and you are left to feel what your new downgraded thyroid is capable of, which isn't much. It's at this point that muscle mass starts to erode if it hasn't already, and body fat starts creeping back on. At this point you also see some of the other warning signs tiptoeing in. Before we talk about each of those in detail, let's examine a couple of ways that Paleo eaters "kick it up a notch" with a real "primal challenge" to squeeze the most out of their beaten down adrenergic system…

Intermittent Fasting

Intermittent fasting is the practice of going long periods without food. It doesn't have to be extreme. In fact, intermittent fasting has a loose definition, and can mean as little as skipping a meal, eating 2 meals per day instead of 3, or eating all your food in a shorter period of time than normal – such as during an 8-hour time period instead of what is more customary – 12-14 hours of eating during waking hours let's say. Or you can go 24 hours without food or longer, all mimicking the supposed long periods our ancestors *might* have gone without food, that *might* have made them healthier. Or not. Ahhh, assumption turned into an eating craze. I love it! Or, more accurately, a non-eating craze.

In short, let's call intermittent fasting "reduced meal frequency." That's usually what it is taken to mean in the Paleo world. Even though studies done on reduced meal frequency typically show hormonal changes with horrendous implications for health (most show an increase in cortisol, crappier glucose metabolism, higher baseline insulin levels, less muscle mass, and more body fat than increased meal frequency – also known as "grazing"), I actually remain somewhat open-minded about it.

I'm open-minded about pretty much anything, as it is so easy to overlook significant details and become too easily seduced by one narrow line of thinking. Anyway, here's the type of study I'm talking about comparing eating frequent, small meals to eating 3 large meals with tons of time in between:

http://www.nejm.org/doi/pdf/10.1056/NEJM198910053211403

Of course, that's not exactly looking at intermittent fasting, but the principles are pretty much the same. Intermittent fasting or IF, undoubtedly increases energy and mental focus (common things reported) and decreases appetite, resulting in weight loss, due to a rise in catecholamines, which usually patterns an increase in cortisol as well (cortisol has been shown pretty convincingly to be the primary root hormonal cause of heart disease, diabetes, visceral obesity – belly fat, and many other undesirables that you can read about in Russ Farris and Per Marin's excellent book, *The Potbelly Syndrome*, Shawn Talbot's *The Cortisol Connection*, Robert Sapolsky's *Why Zebras Don't Get Ulcers*, Ray Peat's fascinating articles at www.raypeat.com, and many others).

You also hear cold hands and feet reported during the fasting period, particularly when practiced during the morning hours. John Berardi talks about this in his book on intermittent fasting, while showing off some really sweet abs and blood tests that show complete metabolic oblivion (low platelets, low white blood cell counts, increased LDL, worse thyroid hormone panels, anemia, testosterone decrease, etc.). Note, weight loss was the cause of this, not necessarily intermittent fasting. But we'll talk about the significance of these icy cold hands and feet later, as this is a common early warning sign of Paleo gone wrong.

Yes, I said earlier that I was potentially interested in intermittent fasting despite some of these very negative implications. There are unforeseen things going on here. I imagine autophagy, an important process of cleaning up metabolic wastes known to increase from exercise and acute bouts of food deprivation, spikes during intermittent fasting. Hey, maybe this trumps the benefits of having lower cortisol with increased meal frequency. Who knows? The wide world of health is too vast to speculate too much here.

But there's simply no question that going long periods without food does work, especially in the short-term, for weight loss – at least it seems to for many people, myself included. It decreases appetite tremendously for me, lowering my natural desire for food intake by anywhere from 500 to 1,000 calories per day if I'm maintaining, say, an 18-hour daily fasting period. In fact, I find the effect to be so strong personally that I absolutely have to eat lots of highly-palatable, calorie-dense refined foods to keep from significantly lowering my metabolism and losing too much weight too quickly. Think buffets.

But what's the mechanism behind this appetite suppression, increased "mental focus," decreased inflammation, etc.? Well, it seems foolish to think that the mechanism is any different than the mechanism that triggers those changes with the consumption of Ephedra or something similar. It walks like Ephedra, it talks like Ephedra...

There are three things about intermittent fasting as it pertains to Paleo that are really scary. The first is that followers of a Paleo diet are already typically eating a low-calorie density, low palatability (the scientific definition), high fiber diet. All of these things DECREASE calorie consumption spontaneously, because all of these things are major appetite deterrents. To that, restrict a macronutrient like carbohydrates and you decrease the palatability even more, and further discourage caloric consumption. The final kiss of death, if the tremendous shock to the nervous system compliments of Crossfit didn't get at ya first, is intermittent fasting.

This recipe is a terrible one. It's like going to a restaurant and seeing French fries served with mashed potatoes, baked potatoes, potato chips, and tater tots. A chef would get fired serving up that combination pretty quickly. Even I, Matt Stone the potato worshipper, with a heart-shaped potato for an official mascot for my website known as the "180 Tatey," who has referred to the Paleo nutrition movement as "just a bunch of tater haters," wouldn't order that one.

Crossfit with lots of rapidly-absorbed carbohydrates = good combo

Whole foods diet with high meal frequency = good combo

Crossfit on ketogenic diet = bad combo

Crossfit and IF on strict whole foods diet = really bad combo

Crossfit, IF, whole foods, Ketogenic = Go ahead and reserve your hydrocortisone for recovery from extreme adrenal fatigue.

Anyway, intermittent fasting, while an interesting intellectual pursuit perhaps for the average health neurotic, is heavy duty stuff. It's powerful. And, like anything that causes dramatic physiological change in the human body, it should be used intelligently. It certainly shouldn't be mandated as part of the biological requirements encoded into our DNA. That's when all this Paleo stuff becomes dangerous. As you'll see later in the book, there are people out there that ran into some very serious trouble. Some are lucky to still be with us.

And the danger with intermittent fasting, just like the danger with strict whole food diets that naturally reduce caloric intake, diets that restrict macronutrients – particularly carbohydrates, doing lots of high heart rate exercise without proper carbohydrate prefueling and refueling (fortunately all the main Paleo leaders are at least supportive of high-carb post-workout nutrition) – can all be linked to increased activity of the adrenal-dominated sympathetic nervous system.

These all seem to have great potential to cause health problems and hasten the basic stress-induced degenerative process – no matter how amazing they may make a person look or feel in the first few months or even year or two with these practices.

Signs and Symptoms of Paleo Gone Wrong

Let's talk about each of the many outwardly signs and symptoms of Paleo gone wrong individually, and cover as many as possible – although there could be many others that I have yet to discover or connect to the metabolic profile induced via carbohydrate and/or calorie restriction (or overtraining) common in the Paleo world.

Once again, let me emphasize that these aren't problems that are exclusive to a Paleo or carbohydrate-restricted diet. You can run into these problems on ANY diet. You can run into these problems just from drinking too much water or not getting enough sleep! There are seemingly infinite paths to producing excessive stress hormones. Whether Paleo was the trigger to your issues or not is irrelevant for this next section. What's more important is identifying the problem and learning how to correct it.

The first and most prevalent is probably the icy cold hands and feet that many experience from having their catecholamines elevated for months and their thyroid toppled in the process.

Cold Hands and Feet

I'm obsessive about cold hands and feet! Because the warmth of hands and feet is an incredible insight as to what is occurring inside of the body. When the hands, feet, and tip of the nose are cold, it is due to reduced peripheral circulation and the constriction of blood vessels in those areas. Peripheral circulation is reduced when stress hormones become elevated. This causes blood to rush from the extremities back toward the internal organs for emergency usage. "Cold feet" is a universal sign of tension, nervousness, or anxiety – all powerful inducers of stress, although they can result from being in a stress-dominated physical state as well. We'll discuss that later.

The thyroid gland is the primary driver of metabolic energy and warmth. Stress hormones are sort of the Kryptonite of the thyroid. They oppose one another, for the most part. The lower the thyroid gland goes due to dieting, emotional stress, nervousness, inflammation, lack of sleep, carbohydrate restriction, overtraining, infection, and so forth – the more prone we are to be dominated by stress hormones throughout the day and night. The low-thyroid, excess adrenal activity combination typically causes the hands, feet, and tip o' the nose to become quite chilly. Sometimes you might feel it in the ears too.

Having cold hands and feet is hardly a health problem, but that's not the point. The point is to see the bigger picture of what is taking place physiologically and hormonally below the surface. And from the research I have done, as well as experimentation and communication with thousands of people all over the globe, all signs point to the physiological state that causes these cold hands and feet being a net-negative to one's health.

That state, is the sympathetic dominant state. While this may sound far out, a simple browsing of the Wikipedia page for the disease of having extreme cold hands and feet (Raynaud's Syndrome) spells it out plainly…

It is a hyperactivation of the sympathetic nervous system causing extreme vasoconstriction of the peripheral blood vessels, leading to tissue hypoxia."

To be clear, and redundant, the sympathetic nervous system is the stress-driven side of the nervous system. While it is always somewhat active, and totally essential to health and function, it's important to know that if your hands and feet are cold, you are most likely unbalanced towards the sympathetic, and the last thing you need to do is engage in more diets and activities that increase sympathetic activity (high protein intake, low-carb diets, intermittent fasting, low-calorie diets, hard physical training).

If your hands and feet were cold to begin with, and especially if they have gotten worse since tinkering around with various diets, Paleo included, you need to run, not walk away from what you've been doing. This is a sure sign that you are not in a healthy state, and need to take action to correct this. Even if you had this problem going into a Paleo diet and lifestyle, this can and should be corrected. Paleo is probably not the right "prescription" for this tendency.

Wiener Malfunction

This doesn't have to mean full-on impotency. It could be something very minor, but still noticeable. If you are a male, you know what I mean. There's 100%, then there's not 100%. And 100%, as a male, is really important. Anything below 100% starts to make you a little mental during sex. And that slight amount of anxiety just produces even more sympathetic activity.

This is a simple issue really. If sympathetic activity decreases peripheral circulation and constricts blood vessels in the extremities (cold hands and feet), and having an erection depends upon maximum peripheral circulation and blood vessel dilation, you are obviously going to see wiener malfunction frequently occurring. That was one of the first early warning signs that I experienced on a lowish-carb diet. Things started running at 80-90% of max power. On a zero-carb diet, or during harsh calorie restriction, I couldn't even spell "boner." As you can see, I spell it perfectly now, even before spell-checking this.

By the same token, creating a condition in the body with more parasympathetic activity usually corrects this in your typical cold hands/feet type of case. As most men have discovered, taking a nap is a great way to restore erectile function, precisely because sleep is the ultimate way to enter into a parasympathetic dominant, restful state (likewise, stress and nervousness has the opposite effect, triggering too much sympathetic nervous system activity and constricting blood vessels in the periphery). But being TOO parasympathetic can cause troubles too, which is why erectile function is usually crappy immediately after a really heavy meal, and why some people, myself included at first, may experience improvements during the first few months on a restricted diet.

In a cold hands and feet type of male, foods that would make a Paleo guru gasp in horror are incredible at restoring lost junk function. Have 4 pints of Haagen-Dazs ice cream, a quart of fruit juice (or soda), and an entire pizza one day. You will likely wake up the following day with levitating sheets (assuming you weren't so hot that you had to sleep bare naked, in the snow angel position), and your love rocket might even hurt. Then the phone will ring. It will be Ron Jeremy. He will want something back and it won't be his hairy back.

There's no question that poor sexual function is a common side effect of bad body chemistry triggered by a poor diet and lifestyle. But getting away from the many pro-sympathetic Paleo commandments can be just what the nurse ordered.

Reduced Sex Drive

While we're on the topic, might as well delve into sex drive too. Sex drive is mostly a matter of metabolic rate and stress hormones once again. The higher the metabolic rate, and lower the stress hormones, generally the greater the production of pro-sex drive hormones like testosterone in males and progesterone in females.

Diets with lower levels of calories and carbohydrates and more animal protein generally work against sex drive. Even just losing weight, which reduces the hormone leptin, will typically decrease sex drive if enough weight is lost – as leptin is the hormone giving the thyroid gland its directions. Sex drive usually returns once the weight is regained.

Basically, when food is scarce – carbs in particular, and stress is high, sex gets bumped further down the Hierarchy of Needs. It becomes less of a priority. It is basic biology. During peak times of year when food is abundant, reproduction takes place. That is why there are mating seasons in nature that generally correspond with times of peak food abundance.
To be truly Paleo, it would be best to keep sex drive minimal all year long on a diet of grassfed meat and raw cabbage, and then feast on carbs in September in the Northern Hemisphere – having sex like a bunny. No thanks.

Loss of Menstruation

Okay okay, it was getting a little bro-ey up there. It's as if I was talking only to the males and leaving you ladies out. But I was thinking about you. I think about you all damn day. Freakin' carbs!

Just as with sex drive being predominantly controlled by the body's perception of "times of plenty," menstruation is under similar influences. Those who fail to menstruate most often are lean, hard-training female athletes. In today's society, we define this lifestyle and physical look as the epitome of health. Oh yeah, not menstruating is like, SOOOOO healthy.

There are other factors that can contribute to a ceased menstrual cycle, but there's no easier way to get there than to lose weight restricting carbs, or fats, or calories, or training really hard, or a combination. Why? Because these things decrease metabolic rate and increase stress hormones. We have built in mechanisms to deter reproduction under these types of conditions – conditions that are not conducive to undergoing a metabolically-expensive pregnancy.

It's an easy problem to fix, but very difficult to fix while following a Paleo diet – especially if carbs are restricted or you are fasting or something like that.

Infertility

Fertility, just like menstruation, is a pretty basic matter of overall metabolic status just like menstruation and sex drive. Females have a lot more that can go wrong hormonally. Generally-speaking, the most important fertility hormone for females is progesterone, as in pro-gestation-hormone.

Progesterone is produced in proportion to the amount of thyroid being pumped out. This causes a higher rate of conversion of LDL, the base molecule of our steroid class hormones, into pregnenolone – which is the hormone from which we synthesize things like DHEA and progesterone.

Stress is antagonistic to that, and carb restriction, low-calorie intake, fasting, hard exercise – these all have the potential to reduce progesterone production to a level that makes conception more difficult, and carrying a pregnancy to term more unlikely. More importantly, reduced levels of progesterone make pregnancy much harder (less progesterone means less cervical elasticity – ouch), and the health of the baby much poorer. More feasting, less fasting. More sleep, less hard exercise. More carbs, less protein. Those are all general rules for the promotion of progesterone production, but it is very person-specific. You never know for sure what a person needs to balance out his or her system. Cravings are usually a pretty good guide. Obey them.

Frequent Urination/Polyuria

While I am sure there is some direct metabolic connection, as I experienced extreme polyuria (urinating frequently, in my case it was up to 5-6 in an hour sometimes) when my metabolism was at its lowest during self-imposed starvation, I don't know the exact mechanisms. I'm sure it has something to do with the interactions of thyroid and/or catecholamines and cortisol and Anti-Diuretic Hormone (ADH), also known as vasopressin. But I'm not aware of how those intertwine.

No matter. The reality is that urinating frequently, with very clear urine that lacks color (taking B-vitamin megadoses doesn't count as having 'color' in your urine), is a clear early warning sign of an impaired metabolism. If you are following a Paleo diet and are having this issue, especially if it has progressed to the point of having to get up to urinate during the night (no it's probably NOT your prostate gland), there is an urgent, no pun intended, need to change course.

You also should notice some correlation between bouts of clear urine and cold hands and feet as well as some of the other telltale symptoms of Paleo Gone Wrong (PGW) like anxiety, dizziness, fatigue, irritability, blurred vision, brain fog, and so on. These are all classic signs and symptoms of an overhydrated state, which occurs more and more easily the lower metabolism becomes – for whatever reason.

I think it's because sugar and electrolyte becomes increasingly scarce in the extracellular fluid when metabolism is reduced – almost purposefully to lower cellular energy production. After all, metabolism begins at the cellular level with the mitochondria's use of what I refer to as the gasoline and spark plugs of the cellular engine (glucose and electrolyte). And when these important fuel sources are scarce, it doesn't take much fluid intake to wash these out – diluting the cellular concentration of these even more. The result is the onset of the many symptoms of hyponatremia/water intoxication and bradycardia. Wikipedia that ish. I also discuss this at great length in another book of mine, *Eat for Heat: The Metabolic Approach to Food and Drink*.

Pay attention to this very important outwardly indicator and respond appropriately. Increasing metabolism is the most important step in overcoming this tendency, but during recovery it's very important to go to great lengths to avoid overhydration. Increasing the intake of calories and carbohydrates and salt and decreasing fluid consumption helps tremendously – especially when it comes to the consumption of solute-free beverages like water, alcohol, and unsweetened coffee and tea. Any plain water consumed should probably have salt and a little fruit juice added to it – mimicking a standard rehydration beverage like Pedialyte or Gatorade – Pedialyte being superior to Gatorade probably, as Gatorade's original formula was altered to be friendlier to the ol' consumer's palate.

Night Sweats

I suspect that this stems from the same condition above, or is at least related somehow. Although night sweats point to a more severe expression. An ex-girlfriend of mine helped show me a lot about the potential downsides of carbohydrate restriction, as I was totally in the low-carb/Paleo infatuation stage when we started dating, but observed her losing her menstruation, having night sweats, almost dying from hyponatremia during a long run, developing deadly shellfish allergies, and developing an autoimmune disease on a low-carb diet – until of course she and I both gave the finger to carb phobia and I watched all of those conditions quickly disappear.

My best guess at explaining both phenomena is that when the concentration of salt becomes too weak in the extracellular fluid, the only way the body can concentrate it is to dump water out. When this happens, even if your bladder isn't anywhere near full, you will feel a sudden urge to urinate. And the urine will be very clear. This can happen during a stressful event, when you have gone too long without eating (including the middle of the night), etc.

The night sweats just seem to be an even more aggressive way of getting water OUT. But there is more to the story, such as the fact that stress hormones peak in the night and early morning (aldosterone, adrenaline, and cortisol – in that general order) and these hormones are diuretic – making you pee whether your bladder is full or not.

Anxiety

Anxiety is a natural mindstate when adrenal activity has become excessive. Anxiety is very common on Paleo/low-carb diets. Drinking excessive fluids really exacerbates it. Catecholamines are probably at the root of the issue, and they can cause obsessive-compulsive thinking patterns, aggression, and other issues to accompany the anxiety.

Irritability

Irritability is also a pretty natural mindstate to be in when catecholamines are elevated. This was one issue that I noticed emerging on a carb-restricted diet. It was fine at first, but over time became a pretty severe issue, especially once I got an idea into my head. I could create a mortal enemy out of thin air it seemed. I can't help but comment on the often militant and aggressive tone that is found in the low-carb sphere, aside from Jimmy Moore. You should see how irate they become when I show them the pivotal role carbohydrates play in lowering fasting insulin and glucose levels and reversing insulin resistance. Scary Taubes!
Again, this is not just a carbohydrate issue. I have experienced this from chronic calorie deficit as well, even when my carbohydrate intake was around 300 grams per day. But problems with carb restriction often have nothing to do with calories. My calorie intake was near 4,000 per day whenever I tracked them during my time on a carbohydrate-restricted diet.

Waking at 4am

Our natural rhythms seem to set 4am as the time to awaken with a surge of adrenaline when things start to become "off." I do believe that this can have something to do with running out of sugar and salt at the cellular level – once again relating to overall metabolism.

Usually there is a strong urge to urinate and feelings of extreme hunger or thirst, rapid pulse, and anxiety. Putting sugar and salt under the tongue at this time is very helpful for taming this adrenaline surge. This is another thing to watch out for and take action to correct.

Lightheadedness

Lightheadedness, or dizziness upon standing, is another classic low metabolism symptom that one can encounter on a prolonged Paleo diet, or a diet of any kind. The subjects of Ancel Keys's famous starvation study at the University of Minnesota all reported this happening and feared fainting and blackouts if they stood up too quickly. This is probably related to bradycardia and hypotension – both telltale low metabolism symptoms. Experiencing starvation myself personally, and extensively reviewing Ancel Keys's work on the subject, is what enabled me to be so capable of spotting the symptoms of a suboptimal metabolic rate – as many physiological and psychological changes that take place when metabolism declines are universal.

Constipation

The creature with the lowest metabolic rate on earth is the sloth. The average body temperature of the sloth is roughly 93 degrees according to what I have read – although I haven't trudged through the jungle poking their buttholes with a thermometer to confirm this. Aside from the obvious undesirable physical characteristics of the sloth, the transit time, or time it takes from food to go from the mouth to the anus, can be up to 30 days!

As metabolism declines, constipation becomes more likely due to the reduced speed at which food travels through the digestive tract. Eating a diet that is high in protein and low in fiber – "low residue" they call it, just seems to exacerbate this constipating effect.

Gastroparesis/Delayed Stomach Emptying

This is a very common problem in the low-carb/Paleo world, and the healthy eating industry as a whole. Basically food just feels like it sits in your stomach like a rock, and the stomach does not empty its contents out into the intestines for way too long. Presumably this delayed time, as well as the delayed time in the intestines that often accompanies it (increased transit time), are an active attempt to squeeze out more energy from the food being ingested.

Get things moving again with a big surge in metabolism (carbs are almost always essential in a case of gastroparesis that develops during carbohydrate restriction, but calories are a greater factor in those who developed the disorder for other reasons, such as reduced calorie density of the diet), and the condition usually improves.

Acid Reflux

This is probably related to gastroparesis/delayed stomach emptying more than anything. But it may also have something to do with reduced gastrin secretion when metabolism is below normal. Gastrin is a hormone that triggers important gastric secretions vital for the proper digestion of food. Acid reflux was something that I suffered from on several different "healthy" diets, worsened the most by excessive hiking because hiking downregulates metabolism (think 2 degree drop in body temperature), but it cleared in just a few days when I raised metabolism via the elimination of macronutrient restriction with increased calorie intake and exercise minimization.

High LDL cholesterol

Blood lipids can improve in the short-term on many diets, Paleo especially. That doesn't mean that these improvements will continue forever. The changes often pattern changes in weight, which go down for a few months, plateau, and then rise again. To really understand LDL, we have to look at some of the basic physiological aspects of the stuff. For that we turn to some of the excellent contributions of Dr. Ray Peat. www.raypeat.com

As far as Peat sees things, LDL is the precursor to the formation of pregnenalone, which later gets turned into our steroid class hormones, sex hormones, DHEA – that kind of good stuff. And metabolism determines the rate in which we convert LDL into these hormones. When we are in the prime of life, we convert at a higher rate. Thus, LDL levels are much lower and our hormone levels are much higher. As we age, this tends to do a reversal. The trick is to keep metabolism elevated the best we can. High LDL is a risk factor for heart disease for the same reason low testosterone and low DHEA are risk factors for heart disease – where LDL is high, you can be pretty sure that LDL is piling up because it is not being converted into testosterone and DHEA.

Sadly, saturated fat, because it causes a transient rise in LDL, has been chastised by the mainstream medical community. Bummer, as that is precisely what gives us the juice to manufacture more testosterone, progesterone, DHEA, and whoop ass.

Anyway, I hope you see the pivotal role of metabolism here. If you see LDL rising on a Paleo diet, you can be pretty sure your metabolism is being negatively impacted and it's time to get your metabolism cranking again.

Low testosterone

Well, we pretty much covered this already I think. But if you would like to see a real life example of a real person who went from an Eskimo diet to a typical 20-something diet built primarily around wheat, and saw LDL levels drop by nearly half while testosterone jumped 120%, you can read this article of mine…
http://180degreehealth.com/2011/03/natural-testosterone-enhancement

Puffy Eyes/Water Retention

This, yet again, is traceable back to metabolic rate. In Ancel Keys's *Biology of Human Starvation*, all the subjects developed severe water retention as their metabolic rate declined. Usually the eyes are puffy in the morning from lying flat on your back all night. Then, during the day, gravity pulls the fluid down towards your hands and feet. Fluid retention is not a good sign. Temporary changes in fluid retention are nothing to be concerned about, but chronic, worsening fluid retention is definitely something to take action to fix – and it could be due to your diet no matter how perfect or biologically appropriate you've been told it is.

Autoimmune disease

Autoimmune disease is something that the Paleo crowd likes to pin almost entirely on gluten. While gluten can trigger an inappropriate inflammatory response in someone with a hyperactive immune system, that doesn't make it the cause. Often, it isn't. I've seen many autoimmune diseases emerge on wheat-free diets, and clear up when wheat is reintroduced, for example.

The theme is definitely reduction in metabolism, which exerts a lot of influence over the thymus gland (thought to be pretty central in the development of autoimmune disease). As Hans Selye's pivotal work on stress showed, the thymus gland undergoes radical change when the catecholamine and glucocorticoids are elevated – a frequent result of calorie restriction, carbohydrate restriction, and other dietary errors. I'm not so concerned with the physiological details though, as all I need are eyes and ears to see that autoimmune disease is a frequent result of a Spartan health regime involving too much exercise, too little food, not enough carbs, lack of sleep, too much stress or trauma, or a combination of several inadequacies.

Just look at the incredibly high rates of autoimmune disease seen with bariatric surgery, for example. Is it because they are eating more wheat on their 400 calorie diets that's causing autoimmunity? I don't think so. Broda Barnes, one of the Godfathers of metabolism, reported that he never saw a single case of lupus develop among his patients – one of the more common autoimmune diseases.

"Throughout my medical career, I have routinely treated each case of lupus I have encountered with adequate thyroid therapy and each has responded satisfactorily without evidence of any involvement of the internal organs. Among the thousands of hypothyroid patients I have treated with thyroid in that time for other manifestations of thyroid deficiency, not one has developed lupus. To be sure, lupus is a very common disease, and yet I have the feeling that thyroid therapy used where indicated to correct thyroid deficiency may act as a prophylactic agent against lupus."
~Broda Barnes; *Hypothyroidism: The Unsuspecting Illness*

Estrogen appears to play some role as well – probably why women are 3 or more times as likely as men to develop an autoimmune disease. But thyroid plays a key role in this as well, as the more thyroid you produce, generally the more of the hormones that oppose estrogen that you produce. This equates to more testosterone in men, and more progesterone in women.

Increased Allergies/Sensitivities

Want to become hypersensitive to gluten and a bunch of other foods? Then cut it out of your diet along with everything else that you might be reacting to.

Not to discredit food sensitivities and allergies. Clearly there are circumstances that warrant removal of certain foods – at least temporarily.

But the root problem in most food sensitivities is the person, not the food. Change the person, eliminate the sensitivity/allergy. I do believe this is a plausible and obtainable goal for a lot of people. I hate to see people quickly eliminate foods from their diet as if it is just no big deal. Restricted diets can paralyze and alienate an entire family from the rest of society. Dietary restriction is a LAST RESORT, not a first line of action. Can ya tell I got a pet peeve with this one?

The etiology of autoimmune disease is probably very similar to the etiology of allergy, sensitivity, and general hyperactivity of the immune system and inflammatory response. There may be another co-factor in why Paleo frequently elicits greater hypersensitivity though – the type of fat consumed in large quantities on a typical Paleo diet.

Paleo eaters often choke down gobs and gobs of Arachidonic Acid (AA) as if it hasn't been shown to directly increase the inflammatory response…

"…research has proven that a high AA diet has the potential actually to change normal immune responses to abnormal, exaggerated ones. A study carried out in 1997 by Dr. Darshan S. Kelley and colleagues at the Western Human Nutrition Research Center in California showed that people on high-AA diets generated four times as many inflammatory cells after a flu vaccination as people on low-AA diets."
~Floyd Chilton; *Inflammation Nation*

Foods highest in AA include eggs, pork fat, organ meats, poultry fat… many Paleo-friendly foods. Many Paleo eaters also consume substantial quantities of nuts and seeds, which contain a great deal of Linoleic acid – a precursor to Arachidonic acid formation with anti-metabolic, pro-estrogen implications. Not good. But even without lots of nuts, seeds, pork, and eggs – just taking in most of your calories as fat ensures much higher levels of Arachidonic Acid intake unless you are hypervigilant about it – but I know of no major Paleo author who has paid much attention to this potentially-important piece of information.

We'll get into this a little deeper later on in the book.

Chest Pain

My recent experiences – which include being able to actually tell a person they have pain in their chest just by analyzing the urea levels in their urine, suggest to me that meat-heavy diets can in fact raise urea levels, and that this is a prominent factor, for whatever reason, in the development of chest pain.

Early on in my blogging and writing career, several people contacted me complaining of pain in their chests. I may not have paid as careful attention to this or assumed it had anything to do with the diet if I wasn't experiencing the exact same thing. About a year into a meat-heavy diet I noticed pressure in the center of my chest. It occurred mostly when I was sunbathing. I would lay there for an hour and then when I went to get up I really felt that pain in the chest. For years this really concerned me, as just eating more carbs, while helpful, didn't eliminate the problem entirely.

Anyway, my own personal solution came from lowering the urea levels in my system by reducing the consumption of pork, shellfish, and several big game fish (which cause urea levels to become elevated – supposedly because they digest much more quickly than other proteins as the story goes, although I can't find much evidence this is true), and eating lighter in the evening – while continuing to eat a diet that was much higher in carbohydrates and lower in meat by percentage of total food intake. I can easily make the problem return by eating meat several times per day.

As voodoo as all that sounds, my personal experience is worth sharing. And if you have chest pains on a meat-heavy diet, it's important to know that you are not alone, it could very well be from your diet, and there are solutions.

Hypoglycemia

This is an endless tangent, and we will talk at great length about carbohydrates and blood sugar regulation later in the book – as this seems to be where Paleos have the most fear and misunderstanding, and stand to gain the most by changing their opinions. But there's no question that carbohydrate and/or calorie restriction can lead to impaired glucose metabolism.

The result is an increasing propensity to experience either true reactive hypoglycemia in response to carbohydrate ingestion, or something that at least mimics the symptoms – most of which can be tied to activation of the adrenal glands, which send blood sugar up and trigger a host of negative symptoms like serious mood changes, shaking, rapid pulse, cold hands and feet, out-of-control appetite and countless others – both minor and major.

While eating a high ratio of protein to carbohydrates has always been the standard crutch relied upon to control the disorder, it is not a solution and makes the root problem that causes the issue in the first place worse. There is another way out.

Bad Breath and Body Odor

Don't know exactly what this is all about, but suspect it has to do with being in more of a catabolic (stress dominant) state. When in a catabolic state, such as coming out of a long fast overnight, it's common to have a pretty coated tongue and strong breath odor. Likewise, when stress hormones become elevated, body odor usually gets very strong. I personally have to cake deodorant on any time I speak in front of a large audience, which also, as expected, makes my mouth dry and hands and feet cold (that's what stress hormones do). But eating a large ratio of meat to carbohydrates can put me there too, particularly if I'm totally sedentary and not doing anything to increase lymphatic flow, blood circulation, oxygenation, etc. Regardless of the scientific reasoning behind it, body and breath odor is certainly a common thing reported from a Paleo or low-carb type of diet. It's certainly not the only cause. Like I said, just speaking in front of a large audience is enough to turn my body and breath odor into foul territory.

Conclusion

This may have seemed like a long list, but it is a very short list. Insomnia, dark circles under the eyes, dry skin, low body temperature, being cold all the time, hair loss, tooth decay or tooth pain, loss of hair on the lower shin, loss of outer part of the eyebrows, hoarseness, heart palpitation and arrhythmia, seizure, migraine, headaches, weight gain, muscle atrophy, chronic fatigue, depression, Raynaud's syndrome…

There are others that I just haven't heard yet I'm sure, or have forgotten. But these are all things that I have, at some point, encountered in people that…

1) Did not have the problem before they started a Paleo diet
2) Developed the problem during their stint on Paleo
3) Had it clear up once they stopped doing Paleo

So these are some real concerns. Of course, you see many positive testimonials as well. And that's great! Yayleo!!! But that's what happens when you have a community that is operating from one narrow point of view, busy defending and promoting their ideologies to save those out there on an even worse diet than Paleo! Paleo is a great rescue religion from overly strict vegetarianism no doubt, and from the Standard American Diet in some cases (but not all – some do much better on a typical American diet than a whole foods diet, especially during recovery).

But again, to be as redundant and clear as possible, this book is about providing a second opinion so that those who are struggling on a Paleo diet understand why, what they can do about it, and see that the logic that they found to be so seductive in the beginning is much more fragile than they originally thought.

So, without further ado, let's viciously attack some of that logic and "sound science" the Paleo community is so proud of. My critiques may come off as being a little harsh and overstated, because in some ways I will be overstating some things. My goal is not to debunk Paleo somehow, which would be a 500-page book with 100 pages of references (I care about keeping this Paleo mania in check, but not that much!!) – but rather present competing ideas in the minds of those reading this that have been brainwashed and are unable to see beyond the ideological rut they are stuck in. Hope it helps. And I hope it is enjoyable, thought-provoking, and well, ya know, makes you have an identity crisis if you've bought into the Paleo version of science.

Or, in 80's movie terms, I hope it helps you "Snap out of it!"

12 Paleo Myths

The problem with any strange and peculiar diet that is radically different from the way the rest of the world eats, is that it's easy, too easy, to disown common health problems that the world is facing. What I'm saying is, if everyone drinks water, then you can blame everyone's health problems on drinking water. Pretty easy to find correlations there. "Hmmm, it looks like nearly 100% of people that have heart disease drink water! Alas, the answer! Hallelujah!"

The same can be said when you condemn enough foods to the point that basically no one on earth is following your diet except you and your small cult following.

People in Asia are getting fatter and have high rates of stroke and stomach cancer? Do they eat grains? Yes! Bingo!!! Paleolujah!
Americans have high rates of heart disease and autoimmune disease? Do they eat lots of wheat, you know, the cause of inflammation? Yes! Boo-yah! Paleolujah!

Similar foolish things are used to support, say, eating a low-carb diet. "Hey, Americans were told to eat a low-fat diet, and after we were told that we became more obese! Carbs are the cause of the whole hackin' obesity epidemic! Can't ya see?"

Of course, this fails to make note of the fact that, despite the government push towards lowering fat intake, Americans still eat one of the fattiest diets in the world. The fattest nation on earth, Nauru, imports big slabs of sheep fat from New Zealand called "mutton flap." Do you really think they could become obese on rice, root vegetables, coconut, and fish? You try it. It isn't easy. You need brownies and mutton flap to do it. High rates of alcoholism don't hurt either.

Anyway, I don't know what that tangent is about or where I was headed with that whole mutton flap thing. I think I just wanted to say "mutton flap." But please do not fall into that trap. I see it everywhere. It's silly.

Now let's begin piecing through 12 myths that I selected to slap around a little. They aren't the only myths. I would have loved to have maybe done a 13th myth entitled "Pork is a healthy food." I could have chosen many more in fact, but I'm just too lazy to do a book called *20 Paleo Myths*. What can I say? I literally live on "Beach Road." It's not conducive to productivity. 12 should be enough to at least get you thinking outside the Paleo box I hope.

A Natural Diet is Superior

We live in a day and age when we are becoming increasingly infatuated with nature. Trust me. I know. I was like the biggest tree hugger ever in my 20's. I once even went out into the wilderness by myself for nearly two months to live off the land. It was like so hunter-gatherer of me.

And it's true that we have definitely strayed a little far away from nature. Our life and diet and everything else is pretty out of sync with what could be called "natural" for our species. While there are some benefits, there are plenty of negative consequences too. Sitting around on my butt in front of the computer for 5-10 hours a day certainly isn't doing my back or posture any favors. Spending most of your time sitting or on your back ain't exactly the key to great bone density for example.

But to have a blind obsession with all things "natural" is to be blind indeed.

Take for example, the cooking of food. Cooking food is not natural. And eating cooked food is not natural for any species. The only species that this could be considered natural for would be humans, but only because we have been doing it for so long. I mean, we were smart enough to do it, so it must be natural in a sense. But it's certainly less natural and less primitive than how other species live.

The Paleo logic assumes that if it is natural, and the diet we are evolutionarily adapted for, it is automatically, without question, the optimal diet. End of story. But an honest look at the cooking of food reveals that cooking food is superior. No matter what you are adapted for. Because it is easier to digest. Cooking breaks the food down so that it can be later deconstructed into its constituent parts – for fuller absorption. All creatures instantly recognize the superiority of cooked food as well, and choose it preferentially over raw food.

While all creatures may be adapted to different diets, all creatures do seem to be instinctually able to recognize the innate superiority of cooked food. Why go out for raw chicken when you've got fried chicken fingers at home? And, as Richard Wrangham points out in his intelligently-written book *Catching Fire*, cooked food is like raw food on steroids for all species. Cooked food yields distinct competitive advantages in size and reproductive rates. No wonder humans fared so well after being the first creature to harness the magical food-enhancing properties of fire…

"We can think of cooked food offering two kinds of advantage, depending on whether species have adapted to a cooked diet. Spontaneous benefits are experienced by almost any species, regardless of its evolutionary history, because cooked food is easier to digest than raw food. Domestic animals such as calves, lambs, and piglets grow faster when their food is cooked, and cows produce more fat in their milk and more milk per day when eating cooked rather than raw seeds. A similar effect appears in fish

farms. Salmon grow better on a diet of cooked rather than raw fishmeal. No wonder farmers like to give cooked mash or swill to their livestock. Cooked food promotes efficient growth... Even insects appear to get the spontaneous benefits of cooked food... Whether domestic or wild, mammal or insect, useful or pests, animals adapted to raw diets tend to fare better on cooked food."

We must ask ourselves whether or not natural truly means "better." In some cases, that may be true. I don't doubt it. In others, it may not be true. Nature is limiting. There is what is natural, and there is what is "supranatural," by definition transcending what is natural in an improved way.

One of the things that helped awaken me from this nature-worshipping coma was reading Roger J. Williams' *Nutrition Against Disease*. Williams was one of the pioneering scientists at the forefront of vitamin research. He did quite a bit of work on B vitamins in particular, and did so primarily by cultivating yeast in a laboratory to study them. Now I know what you're thinking. I'm now going to talk about how awesome megadosing vitamins is. Nope.

I was more struck by what he mentioned about cultivating yeast. When the right blend of nutrients and calories and moisture and temperature collided to create the perfect growing environment favorable to yeast, he could make them replicate so quickly that within days, if laboratory nutrition and environment could've kept pace, the yeasts could have covered the face of the globe. But in nature, there are harsh temperature fluctuations. There is a shortage of nutrients and food supply to feed the proliferation of yeast. Its natural environment keeps the yeast in check, because it's natural for there to be so many damn unfavorable things to deal with in nature.

Likewise, the yeasts were not hardwired with some evolutionary need for hardship, like fasting or calorie restriction or long winters. The easier and more favorable and supranatural the conditions, the better they fared. They thrived in ways that nature never would have allowed.

And cooking food was one of the first ways that we humans managed to create a supranatural environment for ourselves. It no doubt fueled many competitive advantages over other species. As Richard Wrangham suspects, this took us from being merely smarter than the average bear, or ape, to actually starting to develop the impressive cognitive skills that we maintain today. Well, most Paleo advocates wouldn't agree that I personally have impressive cognitive skills, but that's another matter entirely.

When looking at human physiology, we see that, compared to other species of primates and other animals in general, we have very small digestive tracts for digesting and mouths for chewing, weak muscles, and incredibly large, active brains. The cooking of food, because it allowed us to stop diverting so much of our physical resources to digestion, allowed us to develop in other ways. And the more intelligence we developed, the less we needed to run fast, be strong, have fur on our bodies to keep warm, go without food for long periods of time, etc.

With this type of view, the Paleo logic – that powerfully seductive Paleo logic, starts to erode. We can no longer claim that because something was part of the day-to-day life of early humans, that it is automatically superior. That's just not so.

Paleophiles argue that fruits in nature wouldn't have been that sweet, and that we wouldn't have had access to such sweet fruits like we do today. Modern hybridized fruit is much sweeter with less fiber. That makes it better, not worse. I think fruit is the best it's ever been.

You also hear that carbohydrate availability just isn't "natural." We didn't have access to things like fruits and other carbohydrate-rich plants during winter at the high latitudes. I think our 365 day per year carbohydrate access is fantastic for minimizing our exposure to stress hormones – which is the single greatest catalyst to the acceleration of the aging process. These hormones increase as carbohydrate ingestion becomes increasingly infrequent, as a general rule. Stress hormones beat down testosterone, DHEA, thyroid, progesterone – and other pivotal hormones associated with youth, insulin sensitivity, immune system strength, and building and maintaining healthy lean tissue and bone mass.

Hey, some people don't do well eating grains. It's great that we can recognize such things and help people find their way to the right dietary permutation that allows them to live without things like joint pain. But saying that grains are outright inferior for our species borders on lunacy. The result of grain-based agriculture speaks for itself. Grain farming and storage and availability led to the biggest advancement of human civilization in history. It gave us food security like nothing ever had. And rates of reproduction and survival reached new heights on this food that was totally "unnatural" to be eating on a daily basis during a much bleaker era of the past. And I've even found that many people have adapted to grain consumption to such an extent that there is almost a dependency upon eating them for good health. Grains, along with dairy products, are the ultimate human foods in many respects. They are certainly the ideal foods for raising metabolic rate and entering into a low-stress parasympathetic-activated state – two things I have put great emphasis on in my health exploration.

Carbohydrate refining is a totally unnatural process too. And I agree that the nutrient depletion as a result of refining becomes a problem when these foods are consumed in excess, displacing too many nutritious foods. But even the Paleo world acknowledges that rapidly-absorbed carbohydrates are still highly beneficial for glycogen refueling following intense exercise. Muscle growth, exercise recovery, and reduction of exposure to stress hormones are all benefits of rapidly-absorbed carbohydrates ingested in this state. This is another case of the supranatural providing benefits beyond what natural foods can provide.

I'm sure we could go on and on down this path for quite a while. When you realize that natural doesn't always mean superior, it opens up a huge Pandora's box. The beauty is that it opens up true discussion, experimentation, and analysis. Everyone can have a real conversation about the fundamentals of how the human body works. When we can see the context of say, the last example – when it is superior to take in high-glycemic carbs, we have a powerful insight into how the human body works. From that entry point, we can now start figuring out how and when to use such foods, and for whom such foods could be beneficial and why.

Because I can say definitively that the unholiest of the Neolithic foods – white sugar and white flour, can and do serve a vital purpose – and do so despite their potential role in the causation of many modern health problems (yes, the supranatural often does have long-term side effects – but that doesn't mean we can't find a way to take advantage of the many benefits of food processing without the collateral damage).

For example, those of you reading this that are following a Paleo type of diet and suffering from anxiety, cold hands and feet, headaches, blurred vision, frequent urination, dizziness when you stand, sleep problems, etc. – try dissolving a big spoonful of that "deadly" white sugar under your tongue during such an episode without taking in any fluids with it. Or eat a big mouthful of salty, white-flour based pretzels. Odds are it has an immediate palliative effect. You can often prevent major migraines and seizures and all kinds of things with this simple practice – used at the right time. Is it really better to have a seizure than it is to quickly get your body out of its stress state and back into a more hormonally favorable environment? Just because sugar and white flour don't have enough B vitamins in them?

Anyway, that's a deep abyss. But I like to think of things in terms of hierarchy of importance. There are many circumstances where people don't need to be sweating the small stuff (refined vs. unrefined, sucrose vs. honey, grassfed vs. grainfed, raw or cooked, nightshades vs. crucifers) – but need to be focusing on big fundamentals. In today's day and age of intentional deprivation and extreme dieting, I come across a lot more health fanatics in need of a massive surge of digestible calories than anything else to get their metabolism and hormones back in working order. Worrying about the nutritional quality of their diet is something to focus on once normal function is restored.

But we're stressing over the insignificant details with obsessive fervor, often missing the big picture. Paleo is particularly dangerous because the perspective of the movement itself is very narrow. And the psychology of doing what is "natural" with blind faith that natural intervention is always best, is flawed logic that gets a lot of people into really dicey situations with their health. Think bigger. Think broader. And keep your mind open. Just avoiding grains, legumes, and dairy while doing some sprints only solves a very small percentage of people's health problems. There are more solutions out there, some of them in complete disharmony with Paleo dogma. And some of them totally unnatural.

We are Genetically Identical to How We Were 100,000 Years Ago

One of the premises of the Paleo movement is that the human genome developed during the Paleolithic era, and today we share the same genetic "blueprint" of the good ol' primal days. While we are most certainly close to genetically identical to our ancestors, we are 99% genetically identical to most of the other primate species as well. The point is that a little difference makes a BIG difference. Even discovering the tiniest and most subtle differences in our DNA vs. Paleo man would make any arguments that we are identical to our forebears fly out the window.

And we know of such subtle differences. Take something as simple as blue eyes. Humans didn't develop the genetic mutation for blue eyes until an estimated 6,000-10,000 years ago according to the authors of *The 10,000 Year Explosion* – a book about the radical genetic changes that have taken place since the dawn of agriculture. Another of course is the genetic adaptation that humans have undergone that help them digest lactose into adulthood. There are countless others – some discovered, some undiscovered.

The more one sits with the idea that we must obey some dietary laws mandated 100,000 years ago because our genes haven't changed since then gets increasingly flimsy the more time one spends analyzing it. One thing we do know is that the rate of human genetic evolution and adaptation is proceeding at a pace never before seen. Just as the world is rapidly changing, so are we to try to keep up with the runaway train that is modern life.

But more importantly, we are discovering that who we are – our true inherited tendencies and expression, has a lot more to do with things like epigenetics and the intrauterine environment than it does some genetic blueprint. The field of epigenetics has revealed that which genes are turned on and off – in other words how our genes are expressed, in many ways has more bearing on who we are from a health and metabolism standpoint than our actual DNA itself. It appears the last 2-3 generations have the biggest impact on epigenetic triggers of gene expression. Although our actual genetic material may be unchanged, these epigenetic triggers are in place to prepare us for the world that we are about to enter into based on information gathered by the DNA of our parents, grandparents, and great grandparents.

This is a phenomenally cool thing, and is what makes us so highly adaptable. More importantly, it might just make us at least somewhat dependent upon living in at least similar conditions with similar dietary patterns as the last few branches of our family tree. If there's one thing I've seen repeated over the years, it's that dietary extremes don't usually work out very well. I don't know anyone who tried to eat an Eskimo diet and had anything but dismal results long-term. They certainly didn't obtain the kind of health that Eskimos were reported to have, and I don't think it was solely a matter of not eating enough bones or seal blubber or fermented fish. It had a lot more to do with the fact that modern humans are not adapted to such a diet. Isolated peoples that were subsisting off the same diet generation after generation happened to be really well-programed, adapted, and prepared for the nutritional world they entered into.

So epigenetics is a big factor. It is an intricate network of on/off switches that prepares us for the world we are about to enter into. More important to recognize is how wide the variations between two individuals can be in some regards. Yes, we all share very basic biology – not just from one human to another, but all mammals. Some biological themes are totally universal. But there are many fine details and subtle nuances that make us all uniquely individual. Our age, gender, diet history, and other factors make us even more individual in terms of the current state of our health and what needs to happen for us to re-achieve balance.

Because we know so little about epigenetics, it's best to keep an open mind. For all we know, our mom's favorite food might be a dietary necessity with special therapeutic properties that no medical study could ever anticipate! I'm exaggerating a little bit here, but it's the nature of humans to think that we know way more than we actually know. We like to simplify things into condensed theories that are all encompassing, and find comfort in our tidy theories. I find, when it comes to human health and dietary experimentation, no theory holds up. No theory could be vast enough to explain all the crazy, illogical, and unanticipated things that I have witnessed over the years in people's health. But I too used to think it was all so simple. Just avoid white sugar and white flour and you'll live happily ever after! Ah, life was so simple then.

Epigenetics is just a fragment of what can control our actual biological expression. We know, aside from genetics and epigenetics, that mama's uterus has a great deal to do with our hormonal tendencies as well. Now, as disturbing as it is to think about your mother's uterus — and I imagine it's even more disturbing to know that I am thinking about your mom's uterus, it is important. The hormonal environment of the mother appears to communicate in many ways with the fetus — having far-reaching influences over the health risk profiles and metabolism of the kiddo.

We know beyond a shadow of a doubt for example, that if a woman is dieting hard during pregnancy to prevent weight gain, the offspring is typically born with a lower metabolic rate and a much greater chance of becoming obese and diabetic. This makes perfect sense. Dieting sends a strong message of scarcity to the human body, which in turn lowers metabolic rate — lowering thyroid hormone, decreasing progesterone, increasing cortisol, and other unfavorable hormonal changes.

This would then send a signal to the fetus as well that the conditions on the outside world are scarce. Thus, the lil' fella comes into the world metabolically primed to conserve energy, eat a lot when food is abundant and really seek out calorie dense foods, and store a large percentage of any excesses taken in as body fat. And that's exactly what we see. Many things in the modern diet and lifestyle lower metabolic rate, worsened when people then pursue various forms of dietary restriction when they decide it's time to "get healthy."

Wait! There's more! The intrauterine environment has a huge influence over the health and metabolic expression of the offspring. But so does the quality of the mother's breast milk. There are wide variations in the quality of human breast milk from mother to mother. The quality of this milk also has a huge influence over a child's metabolic condition. Human breast milk seems to be becoming richer and richer in linoleic acid (known as omega 6), and lower in short and medium chain saturated fatty acids and cholesterol. Interestingly, omega 6 seems to be predominantly pro-inflammatory and anti-metabolic. The short and medium chain fatty acids seem to have more of the opposite effect, particularly butyric acid (butyric as in butter as in milkfat). Both of these changes tend to favor a lower metabolic rate and higher levels of inflammation. The decreased cholesterol level is also indicative of reduced metabolism. And the more linoleic acid in the milk, well, the greater the number and size of fat cells (the best predictors for one's obesity proneness). The incredible study showing this by French researcher Ailhaud is no longer online of course. FML.

I could obviously go on quite a side tangent here, as we seem to be seeing massive increases in allergies in young kids. The Paleo community is quick to blame Neolithic foods for this heightened state of inflammation, but in theory we should be becoming better and better adapted to Neolithic foods. And kids report allergies to things like eggs, nuts, and shellfish – all perfectly Paleo, as frequently as things like wheat and dairy products. The epidemics of childhood obesity AND heightened inflammation/allergenicity (don't know if that's a word, but you know what I mean – increased proneness to develop allergy) are much more easily traceable to changes in fat consumption (also leading to changes in human breast milk composition) than to increased intake of grains and dairy products. 100 years ago when we had minimal rates of such things, whole wheat consumption, butter consumption, and whole milk consumption were dramatically higher than they are today in the United States. This is true for many countries.

Anyway, breast milk certainly has the ability to alter gene expression depending on its quality. Breast milk is so variable that one woman reported to me that her child was having a bowel movement only once every 4-7 days, but after she changed her own diet to one designed to raise metabolic rate, the child quickly began having 2-3 bowel movements per day. Bear in mind that metabolic rate is the primary controller of bowel transit time, stomach-emptying time, gastrin production, and many other factors related to constipation or lack thereof. Metabolism also has an influence of bacterial flora in the digestive tract.

Yet another factor, although perhaps even more poorly understood than all of the stuff we've covered so far, is how much our own thoughts, emotions, and things like that control gene expression. If there's one sleeper factor that I've seen trump all, it's the power of our perception. Bruce Lipton's *The Biology of Belief* is considered one of the more prominent mainstream books about this, but it is pretty light reading at best. This is a field that we won't be deep into for decades to come I suspect, but we will find it to be significant.

But what does all this have to do with grains, legumes, dairy – that stuff Paleo peeps supposedly didn't eat? And what about the nightshades and things like that, which also contain "plant poisons" designed to deter those attempting to consume? Well, nothing directly really. That's not the point. The point is more that there are so many influences over who we are that have nothing to do with some evolutionary past that took place during the Paleolithic era. So many, in fact, that a simple, broad, human dietary prescription simply cannot be made – certainly not on any genetic basis.

And this of course cuts to the core of my motivation for writing this book. To imprison oneself in a narrow frame of mind about what to eat, is really limiting. And it can be dangerous, as dietary changes are one of the most potent ways of manipulating our physiological function that we have access to. Even a simple prescription like "drink 8, 8-ounce glasses of water per day" is extraordinarily dangerous information if one is led to believe that this will lead to one's peril if not adhered to.

You would be shocked at how many people I am finding who are inducing a great deal of health problems, simply by forcing down the recommend daily amount of water. With the typical human psychology of "more must be better," a simple blanket prescription like that can, and has, ruined lives.

In conclusion, genes are simple compared to the truly unique health situations people manage to get themselves in, which involve everything from deep-seated psychological issues with restraint and restriction when it comes to eating to the fatty acid content of mother's milk and beyond. This is why I constantly find myself antagonizing the dietary Masters of the Universe from the grainstream mainstream to the moist, greasy, bacon-scented seams of the Grok Strap. Yeah, I can be a pain in the ass sometimes. I don't even mean to be or want to be. But somebody needs to throw in some lifelines, giving those that are failing a chance to venture out beyond the narrow perspective they are immersed in.

Each year I become increasingly open to ideas, and create more of a safe-haven of free exploration and experimentation when it comes to health and nutrition. And each year I am completely dumbfounded, confused, surprised, and enlightened by the many insights and revelations that have come from this open-ended exploration.

Just be open. If things are making "perfect sense," take a step back. What you may need to eat or not eat to overcome the health problems you are dealing with RIGHT NOW has nothing to do with genetic mutations that occurred 100,000 years ago, or how many carbs a small tribe gallivanting across Europe had access to. Eating in accordance with our genetic heritage is nothing more than a sciencey-sounding theory with the solidarity of Macaulay Culkin's biceps, and the real world relevance of Corey Feldman's uncle's former co-worker's *Garbage Pail Kids* collection.

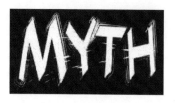

Agriculture Made Us Small and Weak

This is a really dumb argument. I'm not really sure why in the world the Paleophiles would try to bring this up in defense of the Paleo diet. It's just crazy talk. I wonder about their sanity sometimes.

I think it is probably true that early agriculturalists were smaller, with weaker bones, arthritis, and so on. For starters, we probably weren't all that well-adapted to that diet initially. Rapid and sudden changes in diet and lifestyle throughout history have caused dramatic upheavals and transition periods that weren't always smooth from the start. But I don't really think that has anything to do with it.

Rather, as suggested in *Guns, Germs, and Steel*, early agriculture was probably pretty sucky. Agriculture has come a long way since the beginning. Crops have been hybridized again and again to be more palatable and digestible and calorie-dense, as well as drought-resistant, yada yada. Not to mention that up until a century ago or less, famines were common – probably much more common than they were in hunter-gatherer situations where the people had not exceeded the ecological carrying capacity of the land they lived in. Others suggest it was due to the ice age. And there are other hypotheses.

But it HAD to have been something, because the rules of that game have drastically changed. We know that hunter-gatherers today are the smallest little runts on the face of the planet. Agriculturalists, pastoralists, and whatever you would call us (McDonaldists?), are some big brutes in comparison. Try telling a 6'6" Masai warrior to be careful of agriculture because we know it makes people short, as he swills a gallon of milk a day.

And I have my doubts that the members of the NBA were the lucky ones who were raised on grain and dairy-free diets.

Calorie density of the diet and food availability (particularly carbohydrates, sucrose in particular when it comes to height) seems to have a lot more to do with the ability to build large muscles and even height. And neither building muscle beyond a certain point or being tall have any positive associations with longevity or lower rates of degenerative disease. As Paleo researcher Staffan Lindeberg points out, height is usually a positive risk factor for many diseases and a shorter lifespan. Why the Paleo community would repeatedly brag about how fierce and ferocious Paleo man was prior to agriculture escapes me. Current observation of hunter-gatherers refutes the idea that they were large, dominant beast-like men (most hunter-gatherers today are short, and frequently overbellied and undermuscled compared to a typical athlete on a Standard American Diet). And greater size hasn't really been shown by anyone to be a health asset.

From Staffan Lindeberg's *Food and Western Disease*...
"Previously, secular trends of increased body height in the 20th century have been attributed exclusively to improved nutrition, in particular increased

protein intake and less famine. This was called into question already in the 1960's by Ziegler, who showed that the increase in the population's height in England, Japan, Holland, Sweden, Norway, Denmark, USA and New Zealand was strongly correlated to increased sucrose consumption, but not to protein intake. Even observations among Canadian Eskimos point in the same direction. For a 30-year period, body height increased by 4.6 cm among men and 2.9cm among women, while the onset of puberty moved down 2.0 years. During the same period, there was a sevenfold increase in sucrose consumption, while protein intake diminished by 60%."

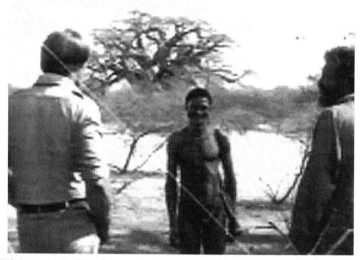

White guys: Dude, you are like really short and scrawny.

Hunter-Gatherer: Yes, I must have gathered too many grains, legumes, and dairy products.

White guys: Yes. We called Loren Cordain and he agreed. We think you should eat more lean meat and wild fruit to get swole bro. Agricultural products made us short and weak. You need protein to get big. Those carbs and dairy will make you small and weak!

Hunter-Gatherer: Makes sense. You white guys are so smart. Hey, you guys go easy on the ice cream once you get back to Nairobi. That stuff will make you tiny I hear. Good thing I've never had it or I would probably be small enough to get hunted down and eaten by a Meerkat.

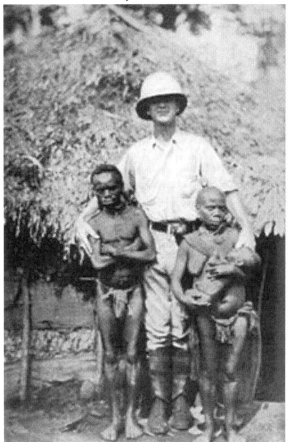

An extreme example... Extremely funny that is – that we think agriculture makes people small and hunting and gathering makes people tall. It's probably more a matter of total calorie intake than anything else – and agriculture, back in the early days, wasn't always synonymous with abundance.

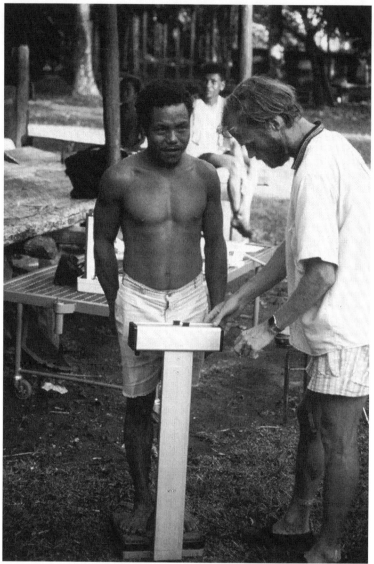

Lindeberg is the guy raised on Neolithic foods… Probably the tallest dude on the island of Kitava the entire time he was there. Why on earth would anyone in the Paleo community insist that agriculture made us small when we are clearly so huge?

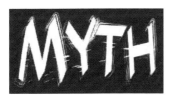

Carbs Cause "Insidious Weight Gain"

In all of the Paleo world, nothing deserves more criticism than the statement and accompanying graphic on page 90 of Mark Sisson's book, *The Primal Blueprint*. In the graphic you see a zone of daily carbohydrate intake ranging from 150 to 300 grams with the label: "Insidious Weight Gain" aside a small cartoon of a chubby man wearing a tie.

This arbitrary zone is described in the following manner…

"150-300 grams a day: Insidious Weight Gain Zone. Most health conscious eaters and unsuccessful dieters end up here, due to frequent intake of sugar and grain products (breads, pastas, cereals, rice, potatoes – even whole grains). Despite trying to 'do the right thing' (minimize fat, cut calories), people can still gain an average of 1.5 pounds of fat every year for decades."

Equally as insulting is the description given for those foolish enough to dare go beyond 300 whole entire grams of carbohydrates a day – still a quite moderate amount by global standards...

"300+ grams a day: Danger Zone of average American diet. All but the most extreme exercisers will tend to produce excessive insulin and store excessive fat over the years at this intake level. Increases risk for obesity, Metabolic Syndrome, and type 2 diabetes."

This, in all the world of nutrition and health, is some seriously revolting bullshit.

Now if I were Mark Sisson, and I lived in Malibu, CA – I too probably wouldn't bother to travel much. I mean, why travel if you live in Malibu? It's a nice place. David Lee Roth couldn't have been far away from Malibu when he filmed the "Wish They all Could be California Girls" video. Can't be too far from Baywatch either. Why go out for Schnitzel when you've got Hasselhof at home?

If he did travel, he might notice that most of the other places in the world have much leaner citizens. In places that I have travelled to, like Vietnam (or Cambodia, Nepal, Japan, Laos, Thailand, Dominican Republic, Honduras), obesity is more or less nonexistent. I don't recall seeing a single person with what could be considered a problematic amount of body fat in say, Vietnam.

And I, at a whopping 5'9" 170 pounds with about a 33-inch waist at the time, remember one day when I was hanging out on the beach at Cat Ba island in North Vietnam. I was laying around on the beach drooling. Doing my thing. My favorite pastime. There were maybe 10 other people at the beach. And along came a small boat with about a dozen young men about 20 years old.

The boat came over near the shore, dropped anchor, and the boys all jumped out and swam to shore. They were running around like goddamn apes, jumping over each other, putting sand down their Speedos and giggling, wrestling, racing each other, and in typical Vietnamese fashion – making absurd amounts of noise, totally oblivious to anyone around them.

After a minute or two of this they got bored and did what any Vietnamese person would do to a complete foreign stranger – run over to me and start talking loudly in my face and touching me without even introducing themselves. They pinched the tiny half inch of fat or so around my waist and laughed, calling me fat. Then the sort of Alpha of the group challenged me to a swim race – to which I knew I was doomed (I'm like the worst swimmer ever – my 9-year old niece can outswim me easily).

I was quickly obliterated in the wake of this "some young guy." Then the boys laughed, came over to play with my tiny body fat stores once more, and then swam back to their boat – never to be seen by me again.

The point here is that not only were all of these boys lean and energetic, they looked at me like a novelty because I had some body fat. And we're not talking a lot of body fat here either. I couldn't have been much over 12-13% body fat at the time. It was a novelty because it was so rare, and what is the composition of the Vietnamese diet? Do they eat more meat and fat and less carbohydrates on a grain-free "Primal" diet? Did these guys wake up to bacon and eggs? Were they headed off to have some Paleo pork ribs and non-starchy vegetables for lunch? Of course not. The Vietnamese diet, like most diets of the 7 or so billion people on earth, is grain-based and much higher in carbohydrates by percentage of total calories than the Standard American Diet referred to by Sisson.

Now I've got no problems with meat and fat, and I'm not recommending or condoning a truly low-fat diet. I've seen lots of people suffer from eating a diet that is too low in fat. It's a great way to become asexual and depressed in my experience, due in large part to underconsumption of calories – a virtual guarantee when eating fat-free cardboard.

But I've seen the same negative results with even mild carbohydrate restriction as well – in myself and in others that have come to me to share their story over the years. That's a primary motivator for writing about all this. Trust me, I don't revel in being hated by the Paleo community or being banned from websites like Mark Sisson's www.marksdailyapple.com or Richard Nikoley's www.freetheanimal.com.

The point is simply that making a broad, sweeping generalization about carbohydrate intake that has 5 billion living contradictions to it, is just plain wrong. It is, like the title of this book suggests, a Paleo myth.

In reality, there are no epidemiological studies that show this type of correlation between carbohydrate intake and obesity. Most show the opposite in fact, with the countries that have the highest access to meat and fat (and food in general) being the fattest. While the leanest places on earth – large portions of Asia and Africa, subsist on grain-based diets built around staples like rice, millet, teff, wheat, legumes, and so forth.

Sisson claims that the fattening offenders are: *"breads, pastas, cereals, rice, potatoes – even whole grains."* Yet, in the United States over the past century, there has been a decrease in the consumption of grains, corn, and potatoes that has accompanied the large rise in average bodyweight.

Changes in the American diet from 1909 to 1999, as reported by the USDA (and reported in the *Encyclopedia of Healing Foods*):

- Consumption of whole milk dropped 49.8%

- Consumption of skim milk increased 57.8%
- Consumption of butter dropped 72.2%
- Consumption of margarine increased 800%
- Consumption of shortening increased 275%
- Consumption of lard and tallow dropped 50%
- Consumption of salad and cooking oil increased 1,450%
- Consumption of fruit increased 29%
- Consumption of vegetables increased 15.6%
- Consumption of potatoes dropped 23% (of fresh, unprocessed taters, it fell by 73%)
- Consumption of grains dropped 30.6% (corn by 50%, wheat by 30%)
- Consumption of pork dropped 19%, eggs dropped 13.5%, beef increased by 22%, poultry increased 278%
- Consumption of legumes and nuts increased 37.5%
- Refined sugar and syrup consumption increased by 74.7%

Note: If you want to have a serious conversation about doing something truly "unnatural," picking on grains and dairy is ridiculous – especially seeing how much the consumption of them has dropped as basically all degenerative diseases have risen. But squeezing oil out of corn and soybeans and hydrogenating it and increasing the consumption of it by roughly 1,000% – well, that's a different story.

Note 2: Overall carbohydrate consumption fell from 57% of calories to 46% of calories.

This is similar to the dietary changes seen in places like the Pima Indian Reservation during their transition from lean to the world's most obese and diabetic people…

> "Over time, the Pimas' diet gradually shifted away from wheat, beans, squash, and produce gathered from the desert and began to resemble that of the rest of the country. Beginning in the 1930's, federal and state programs provided high-fat foods such as bacon and cheese. After WWII, the U.S.D.A. expanded the types of foods supplied to include milk, canned meats, fruits, vegetables, and dry cereals. Gradually traditional dishes such as cholla bud stew…posole."
>
> "Researchers at the NIDDK in Phoenix have estimated that the traditional Pima diet took about 70 percent of its calories in the form of carbohydrates, 15 percent in protein, and 15 percent in fat. By the 1950's the proportions had changed to 61 percent carbohydrate, 15 percent in protein, and 24 percent in fat. In 1971 it was 44 percent carbohydrate, 12 percent protein, and 44 percent fat – a tripling of the fat content."
>
> -Robert Pool; *Fat: Fighting the Obesity Epidemic*

I did come across one study that showed a strong connection between weight gain and potatoes. Of course, the potatoes, in the modern American diet, are consumed as potato chips and French fries – which, by percentage of calories, are only 45% potato or so – the rest fat. And what kind of fat? Polyunsaturated fat primarily from soy and corn oil – a type of fat known to increase inflammation and decrease metabolic rate (both major factors in obesity). In rat models, the more polyunsatured fat they were fed, the fatter the rats got with each generation until they were all obese after several generations. A good database of references to back up some of these claims can be found at www.raypeat.com, or www.andrewkimblog.com, or this really good summary…
http://pranarupa.wordpress.com/tag/pufa/

And many others. Okay, back on track…

Actually consuming potatoes – like baked potatoes or boiled potatoes or mashed potatoes, reduced their fattening effect. In other words, the more potatoes in the potato, the less fattening it was. Get 60% or more of your calories from potatoes and tell me how fat you get doing it. In the right context, the potato is one of the most excellent foods for improving body composition. The potato's satiety index is one of the highest of any known foods – perhaps because taters raise the appetite-crushing/metabolism boosting (eat less, burn more) hormone leptin as much or more than any other food on a calorie for calorie basis. Okay, enough about taters. Love them things though. Don't be no tater hater!

I could go on for an entire book about the false belief that the carbohydrate is inherently fattening, or that a diet with more than 150 grams of carbs will cause insidious weight gain. In fact, in the second half of 2011 I lost about 15 pounds, and I did so without ever eating, to my knowledge, less than 300 grams of carbohydrates in a single day – much less under the 150 gram "mark."

For now let's just say what Mark Sisson's claim about carbohydrate intake is… It's retarded. It's disgraceful. It's wrong. It's inaccurate. There is absolutely no scientific or observational validity to it. It's just plain crap, and, despite many of the wonderful health principles coming out of the Sisson camp, this one idea is enough to single-handedly make a mockery of the man who made the mistake of writing it. I've written some really dumb stuff too, but eventually I always correct myself when I have new insights that make me capable of seeing my mistakes. I hope Sisson can think his way out of this one, and come clean on it. He's made a few feeble attempts, but could definitely try harder.

And I apologize for my disrespect to the man, but this, to me, represents the absolute worst of the crazy health and nutrition-obsessed world that we find ourselves in in 2012. I even recognize the possibility of using carbohydrate restriction as a potential dietary therapy for certain situations. But there is a huge difference between writing a book which asserts that carbohydrate-restriction "might" be of some benefit, that our ancestors "appeared" to be healthier by many yardsticks and that their diet "may" have had something to do with that… so you "could" potentially try it for yourself and see if you notice any improvements…"

… And a book which makes wild and false claims that if you eat more than a certain amount of carbohydrates, it is dangerous and will inevitably lead to weight gain.

The latter scares people, creates unnecessary and dangerous phobias, creates a lot of anxiety and social awkwardness, and who knows what else. Anyway, I've seen enough people damaged by it that couldn't seem to get out of the hole they were in due to the powerful ideological component of the Paleo diet (the idea that carbs are bad is ridiculous, one of the best documented primitive groups of people on earth get over 2/3 of their calories as carbohydrates each day – the Kitavans), that I couldn't help but put this Sisson garbage where it belongs. I hope it brings some sanity to the people that read this who are suffering from the carb-phobic propaganda they've been exposed to.

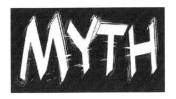

Insulin Resistant People Store More Glycogen

This isn't some major prevailing myth in the Paleo community, or something that is even talked about much. But as you'll see, Art De Vany had a little glycogen slip in his new book, and I'm so interested in glycogen storage that I couldn't help but write about it. Anyway, follow along peeps…

Glycogen is some important stuff. In fact, I think a lot more research should probably go into glycogen synthesis, storage, release, and usage. When you start to look at diabetes and insulin resistance-related research from a glycogen point of view, it paints a completely different picture than what you hear in low-carb influenced spheres of nutrition. Or even what is believed by the mainstream, which seems to be thinking of diabetes in a similar way more and more each year (unfortunately).

Glycogen is stored carbohydrate. When you eat a meal, you produce glycogen synthase, which helps to convert carbohydrate into its storable form. Then, with the help of insulin glorious insulin, glycogen gets packed away for later use in muscle and liver tissue. Glycogen is, essentially, rocket fuel for muscular work. And it is very important. When glycogen stores are low, metabolism tanks, athletic performance tanks, and fat burning comes to a standstill – a phenomenon summarized in Loren Cordain and Joe Friel's book on exercise by the phrase, "fat burns best in a carbohydrate flame." Strangely, most of the Paleo community thinks that to burn fat, glycogen levels need to be depleted. Oops.

An extreme example of low glycogen levels is what is referred to in extreme endurance athletics as "bonking." The body is basically useless at that point. The tank is empty.

And while I think one of the Paleo Godfathers - Art De Vany, is a pretty cool guy with some great ideas – especially on exercise, I take serious issue with one of the major errors he makes in the book he recently released called *The New Evolution Diet*. In the book, Art says:

"He or she will look somewhat husky, because metabolic syndrome causes fats and glycogen, a form of sugar, to build up in muscles, giving them a bigger look."

He is essentially saying that one of the hallmarks of insulin resistance and metabolic syndrome is an EXCESS of stored muscle glycogen.

That sounded fishy to me. Over the years I have come to think of insulin resistance, prediabetes, and type 2 diabetes as being problems with the storage and usage of sugar. A normal, healthy person can eat a big, whopping load of carbohydrates. I often sit down and eat up to 300 grams in a single sitting myself (of total carbohydrates). And when I or another insulin sensitive person eats a big load of carbohydrates like this, insulin rises swiftly and the carbohydrate is rapidly shuttled into the muscle and liver in the form of glycogen. Meanwhile, the levels of glucose in the bloodstream hardly change. It is true that my blood glucose rarely travels above 100 mg/dl no matter how many carbohydrates I eat. Getting sugar out of the blood quickly is referred to as "glucose clearance," and in my view is very revealing in terms of one's "glucose metabolism fitness level."

And it's pretty easy for most people to improve. In fact, a type 2 diabetic that I've worked with for only 3 weeks now has already seen a 1-hour postprandial blood glucose reading only 2 points above her fasting level at about 130. On the first day she was at 359 mg/dl after a meal to give you an idea at just how rapidly improvements can be made.

I view people with impaired glucose clearance as those who can't clear all the glucose precisely because it isn't being stored properly, causing sort of a traffic jam. The result is high levels of sugar in the blood and low levels of sugar in the muscle cells themselves – causing a general feeling of being depleted (low energy, fatigue) and a decrease in metabolic rate when muscle carbohydrate levels aren't full.

If it were true that insulin resistant people really do have increased glycogen storage and their muscle cells are totally overflowing with sugar, that would have provided a pretty good lashing to the way things work according to what I've been led to believe. So, after throwing Art's book across the room and shouting expletives kind of like Yosemite Sam, I figured I better look it up to see why Art would say such a thing.

So I quickly Googled something like, "insulin resistance and glycogen storage." And, within minutes, I was ripping through a pretty clear-cut and straightforward study showing that Art's claim about glycogen stores being higher was totally bass ackwards. In fact, in the first study I read it was shown that glycogen synthase was reduced by 60% in the insulin resistant subjects vs. the normal controls in response to a meal. And overall glycogen stores were reduced by about 20%.

http://www.ncbi.nlm.nih.gov/pmc/articles/PMC1924794/

Along with that decrease in glycogen storage was an increase in the percentage of fat supplying energy. Think about that for a minute. The supposedly desirable (according to most in the Paleo realm, such as Art De Vany, Mark Sisson, and Loren Cordain) metabolic condition of burning fat for fuel was a characteristic of someone with insulin resistance. Burning carbohydrates as a primary source of fuel was more typical of a healthy, insulin sensitive person. This is why I put more focus on how to restore the proper storage and usage of glucose, rather than encourage activities that increase dependence on fat as a fuel source (like low level cardio, sedentarism, stress, and eating lots of fat/low-carb).

Anyway, I think Art must have been basing this off of the pervasive low-carb rumor that those with insulin resistance suffer from the disorder because they've simply eaten too much carbohydrate. In that fantasy world, the cells of diabetics become saturated with all that sugar they eat, and the muscle cells just won't accept any more sugar. When glucose in the blood goes to be stored, the muscle cells respond like the kids on the bus when Forrest Gump was trying to find a seat. "Seat's taken!"

Forrest Gump-like indeed, as this would be the way that someone who is a little special would view glucose metabolism. It's just, like many things in the Paleo realm, out of touch with reality.

I don't propose to know all the ins and outs of glucose metabolism. No one knows or fully understands it. But we can rule out the version of science that circulates through most of the Paleo realm. This sugar tank isn't full. The tank itself is smaller. And because the engine isn't burning sugar well the poor hunk of junk has gotta run off motor oil instead. Being insulin resistant sucks, not because there's too much sugar, and insulin is so high that fat can't be burned for fuel. That just isn't so. A more accurate depiction of what's really going on might be to say that those with insulin resistance don't have the luxury of burning glucose for fuel at the same rate of those that are insulin sensitive. Their bodies are too busy converting that glucose to fat and using fat as a fuel source.

A more appropriate way to look at how to improve our epidemic of insulin resistance is to look at real, factual information on what the defects are and how those defects can be prevented or improved upon. And Paleo, because it is in its own separate universe aside from science (because of the moronic need to send every scientific truism through a caveman approval process – rice increases glycogen storage, but Grok didn't eat it... Grade: F), is actually impairing the nutrition world's progress towards using dietary manipulation with greater precision.

The trend, thank Grok, is for Paleo to incorporate more and more real science and real life responses to certain practices. One trend in particular that is starting to catch on, is eating large amounts of carbs as a "re-feed" or during the post-workout time frame. Refilling glycogen every few days while following a low-carb diet is a massive improvement over being low-carb all the time. There is indication that depleting glycogen stores pretty thoroughly and then going crazy on carbs causes an impressive glycogen supercompensation effect. http://www.ncbi.nlm.nih.gov/pubmed/3698159

Glycogen is the most depleted after very high intensity exercise (recommended by Paleo, even though Paleo people did mostly endurance exercise to the detriment of their health and physiques), after prolonged periods without food (recommended by Paleo), and after long periods of carbohydrate restriction (recommended by Paleo). So if insulin resistant people store less glycogen, and that seems to be one of the root problems with the disease, some of these practices

MAY have a use – barring the many potential unintended negative consequences of some of these practices (and ignoring the fact that most people shouldn't be turning their eating into a science experiment – but should probably just eat, relax, and be normal members of society with the minimum amount of diet mindfulness for mental, social, and physical health – I mean, do you know a soccer mom whose kid complains that she is NOT talking about food enough? In other words – we are already collectively thinking about what we eat way too much).

But this gets back to my primary point in doing a critique of the Paleo movement in the first place. Paleo is getting better by becoming more scientific and a lot less Paleo. The less Paleo it becomes the better it gets. The sooner that the Paleo movement goes, wait for it… "extinct," and turns into something intelligent, and used intelligently, the better. We shouldn't have to ignore reality and pursue something ethereal and poorly-strategized to prevent and correct health problems. My vision for the medical use of nutrition and lifestyle manipulation in the future is much greater than what is going on in the Paleo community. It is very possible to use a great deal of exactitude and precision with dietary and lifestyle manipulation to achieve an intended hormonal response/adaptation.

Suffering from adrenal burnout and low thyroid? Okay, then eat a ton of calories, particularly sugar, starch, fat, and salt – pizza and ice cream with a large root beer – and you will quickly be thrust into a parasympathetic dominant state, drooling in a state of deep relaxation with a substantial rise in body temperature with warm hands and feet characteristic of being in that state. With the condition of excess sympathetic activity, squabbles over insignificant things like casein or micronutrient content or whether or not our ancestors ate it become not just irrelevant, but highly distracting. More like a giant mental barrier. Like what the Green Monster is to fly balls to deep left.

Back to glycogen... I really do think that increasing one's stored carbohydrate tank could be one of the most pivotal changes one can undergo in overcoming the basic metabolic syndrome profile – a primary risk factor for most of our degenerative diseases. And doing this seems to boil down to the basic idea of emptying the tank, and refilling the tank, and emptying the tank, and refilling the tank. In other words – giving the body strong motivation to increase the amount of reserves.

But that is just one limited viewpoint. To keep cortisol minimized, the primary hormone implicated in insulin resistance, it might actually be better to keep glycogen full ALL the time to minimize stress with frequent carbohydrate feedings.

So yes, although there is a ton of research refuting the idea that depletion of glycogen through intermittent fasting, reduced meal frequency, calorie or carbohydrate restriction, or high intensity exercise will yield improvements in health, insulin sensitivity, or body composition (most, like the ones below, show increases in cortisol and crappier glucose metabolism) – there is enough out there to at least remain open about it.
http://www.ncbi.nlm.nih.gov/pubmed/17998028
http://www.nejm.org/doi/pdf/10.1056/NEJM198910053211403

Yes, that's right. Even though I have seen people completely ruin their health and achieve quite amazing states of extreme stress (sympathetic nervous system activation) from carbohydrate restriction, intermittent fasting, and high intensity exercise – to the point of having discoloration in their fingertips on a 73-degree day in Orlando, I remain open about their usage.

We should be open about everything. If something can elicit a powerful response and hormonal change, and is as simple as eating on a different meal schedule, (ain't exactly chemotherapy), then we should look into what health problems might be alleviated from that change. We should look openly at the medical use of nutrition and work together – acknowledging both the short-term and the long-term, the positives and the perils. And get better as we move forward without clinging to one and only one cultish belief system.

Because no Paleo leader would ever recommend sitting around and eating ice cream all day.

And that's unfortunate, because that's exactly what some people in some metabolic conditions need. That might be the perfect thing for a person with anemia, low white blood cell counts, low platelets, anxiety, and/or cold hands and feet to do. It could be great for someone who is underweight and suffering from Bacterial overgrowth of the small intestine. It could be awesome for a young kid who is failing to thrive, as ice cream has an almost identical macro and micronutrient profile to human breast milk.

I hope you see what I'm getting at here. I'm merely calling for an honest look at what something like intermittent fasting does. Then you take a look at an individual and their basic symptomology and try to figure out if the hormonal changes seen with intermittent fasting would represent a positive change for that individual, or a negative change for that individual. As it currently stands, the Paleo community assumes that cavemen did this, and that their health was made better by doing it, and that because our ancestors did it we absolutely must have some kind of genetically determined need to do it too or we will become ill.

Even having to go through the exercise of trying to "refute" that idea is tremendously painful and tedious for me, for the same reason that writing an entire book about why 2+2 does not equal 5 would be a painful and tedious exercise. I simply don't understand why we have to stoop to such a low level of intellect to discuss health. Or, get so wrapped up and attached to certain practices.

"Wow, intermittent fasting helped me lose 50 pounds and my arthritis is gone, and I HATE Matt Stone because he said bad things about intermittent fasting!"

But the reality is that if something is powerful enough to change human physiology that much, it is perfectly capable of doing great harm. And it does do great harm. It does great good. It depends entirely on the context and the person intermittent fasting is interacting with. We should learn how to do it better – not just bring up more and more studies about how amazing it is in rodent studies and then tie it to some nebulous unknown about what some 24-year old male had to do 90,000 years ago because the weather was too crappy to go out and hunt that day. All this does is create psychological entrapment for those who immerse themselves into the Paleo subculture – sometimes to the detriment of their health.

Crap, there I go on another tangent. Sorry.

So yeah, glycogen. It's good. A hallmark of health. We want more of it. And Art De Vany who thinks that insulin resistant people look puffy because they have more glycogen than he does is very confused. Art, with his practices of occasional fasts, hard exercise, carb restriction, and a feast from time to time – probably has far greater glycogen storage than an insulin resistant person. And is healthier for it. It's a minor "Paleo Myth," but because I happen to think that glycogen is particularly interesting when it comes to metabolic syndrome, I would hate to see this myth perpetuated in the Paleo community. I would rather see them putting more emphasis on massive, periodic refeeds for achieving glycogen supercompensation like that used in the bodybuilding and fitness industries – for better health, recovery, performance, maintenance of metabolic rate, stress hormone reduction, and everything else in between.

But no matter what, it's pretty clear that EVERYONE should probably be having at least a few carbohydrate feasts per week, regardless of what seasonal availability was in the Arctic circle during the late Paleolithic era. I still prefer to have several carb feasts per day, and continue to suspect that constant carbohydrate availability was a practice that every culture on earth adopted because of its awesomeness, not its foolishness. Eating carbs all day sure as hell helps the insulin resistant people I work with.

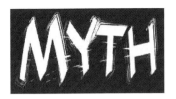

Hunter Gatherers Had Sexy Bodies

By sexy body I basically mean well-muscled and lean. Of course, that is an arbitrary definition, but so is Mark Sisson's sickening love fest with Grok being like a "Decathlete" and Grok's lady friend being a "hottie."

Most of the secrets on how to develop muscle tissue and increase leanness – develop a "sexier" body by modern standards, have already been solved by exercise physiologists and the fitness industry. There are certain physical stimuli that produce muscle development – mostly high-volume, hard muscular work in unfavorable leverage positions in the 8-12 rep range with minimal rest in between sets to prevent full ATP restoration. For growth, calories must be kept high, with an emphasis on carbohydrates and protein while keeping fat at moderate to low levels – but not so low as to deter calorie intake or affect testosterone levels unfavorably. While different people seem to do better with a certain macronutrient ratio – with nothing fully universal, grains and dairy almost always factor into that equation – starches seeming to perform better than sugars (grains being superior to fruits and vegetables is fair to say). This is partly due to the increased calorie density and palatability of grains and dairy products, which make it much easier to get into an anabolic, muscle-growth state.

As far as getting and staying lean, most success stories come from fitness enthusiasts that eat frequent meals of rather bland starch and protein combos, combined with all kinds of advanced diet cycling techniques to prevent metabolic downregulation. But there are obviously multiple paths to the same destination.

We can talk about the fine details all day long, particularly the getting lean part as the world's leading obesity researchers are still pretty clueless about how a normal overweight person can change his or her body fat levels on a permanent basis. The point of the matter is, humans know about and are achieving more with aesthetic physiological change than ever before in human history. Even just the last 100 years has seen dramatic advancements in the science of sports physiology, muscle development, etc. And the result has been giant leaps in what people have achieved physique-wise.

Yes, performance enhancers like steroids, amphetamines, growth hormone – those are responsible for many changes. But even the major differences between old school bodybuilders like Charles Atlas and Eugene Sandow and how they compare (well, they don't compare, really) to modern, all-natural, steroid-free fitness and figure athletes is remarkable. Just like in any technology or sport over the past century, where we are at now is well beyond where it once was even just a short time ago.

And the bodies of today's natural bodybuilders, fitness models, athletes??? WAY beyond anything seen amongst the remaining tribes of hunter-gatherers around the world – who live and eat more closely to our Paleolithic ancestors than anyone on earth.

Anyway, it just doesn't make sense to try to glorify and mimic the hunter-gatherer for his or her aesthetics when much of what hunter-gatherers did flies in the face of what we know about aesthetics today. But worse, we have no reason to believe that hunter-gatherers did have aesthetics that are in any way remarkable – especially for the amount of physical activity they most assuredly were engaged in. In fact, in the rest of this short chapter, I will put up some pics of hunter-gatherers looking pretty pathetic compared to modern athletes – who have superior training and a superior diet and therefore have superior hormonal excellence and the freakish aesthetics to match. Hopefully you will at least acknowledge that the Paleolithic era and modern hunter-gatherer tribes may NOT be the ultimate place to turn to for physique development, but rather you should be turning to people like Kevin Weiss and Martin Berkhan and studying the science behind their methods…

Bryan Clay – Decathlete

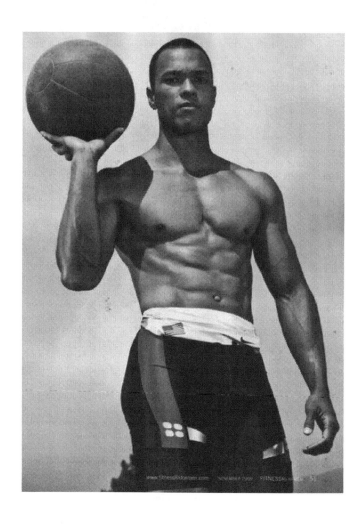

Hunter-Gatherer (Kind of like the Javelin?)

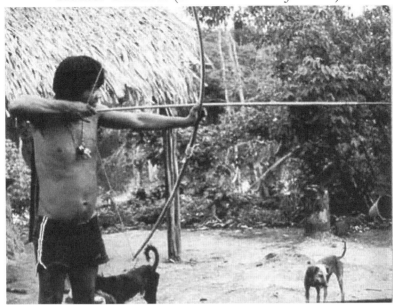

Young Gymnasts

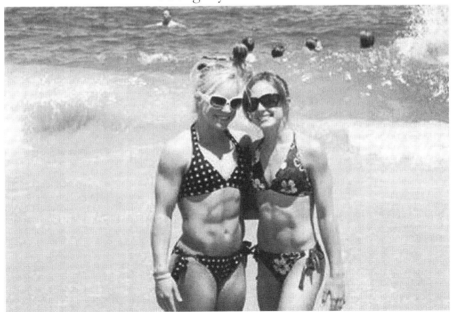

Lost Amazonian Tribesmen and Women

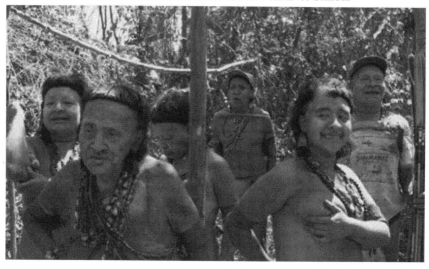

Ernestine Shephard (age 74)

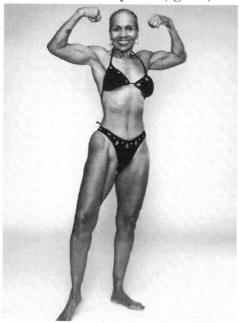

Old Hunter Dude

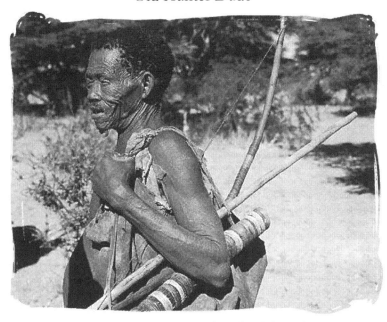

Kevin Weiss (100% Natural drug-free bodybuilder, loves Oreo Cakesters)

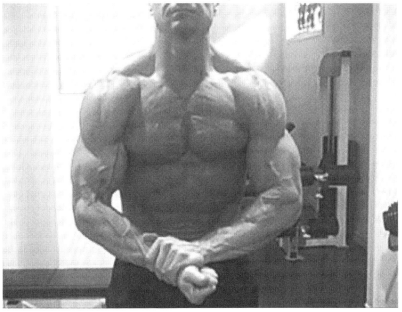

Here's a video featuring Weiss and his colleague Scott Abel (the world's leading expert in physique development if you had to narrow it down to just one person) describing one of the cutting-edge supplements he uses to get in this condition: http://youtu.be/LrF_UjhdxWg

And here's a collection of other hunter-gatherers eating Paleo diets and living Paleo lifestyles around the world…

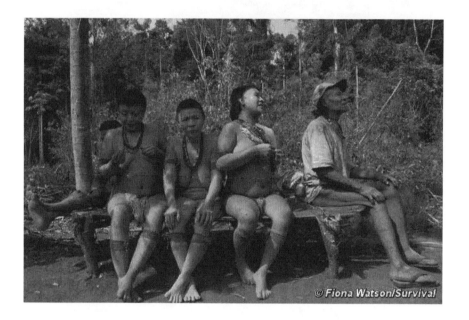

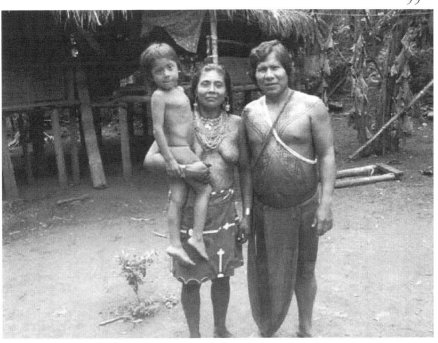

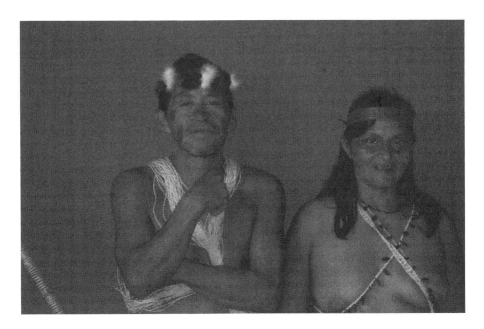

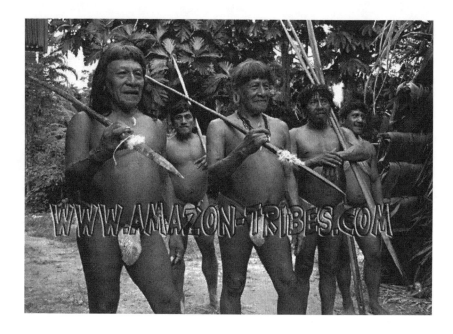

Here is a rare snapshot taken of an isolated tribe that just came into contact with other humans for the first time ever…

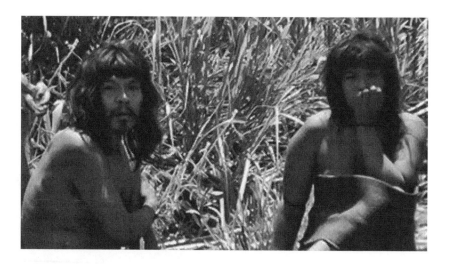

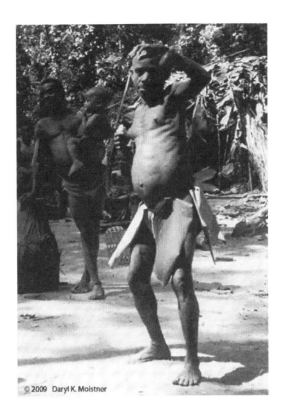

And please let's not forget the totally unenviable physiques of the Tarahumara Indians that run ultramarathons regularly as cataloged in Christopher McDougall's absolutely ridiculous book about how we are "born to run" or something like that...

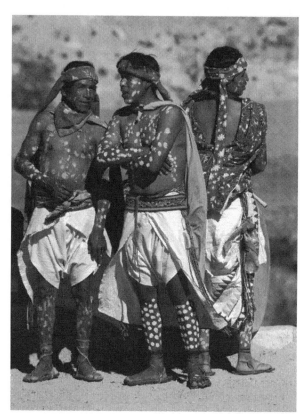
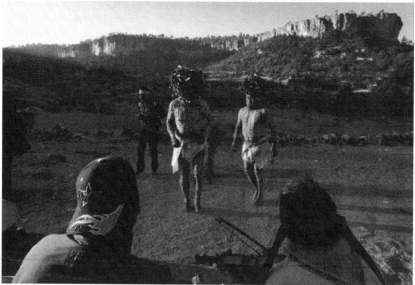

Martin Berkhan Flexing (No jogging required for this physique)

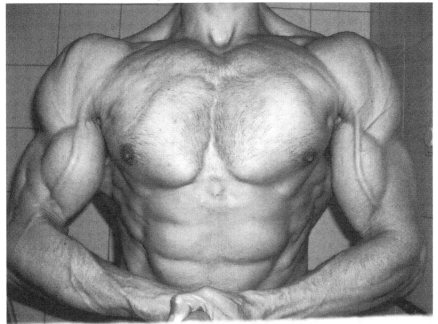

Martin Berkhan Preparing to attack an entire Cheesecake Like a Badass

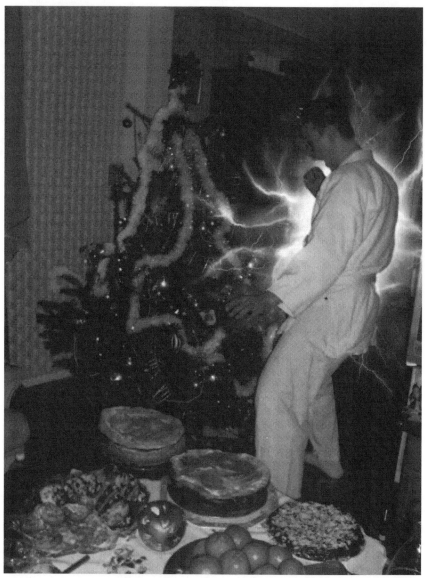

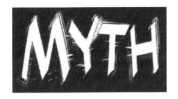

Carbohydrates Cause Insulin Resistance

It is a pervasive myth in the low-carb and Paleo worlds, two worlds that are way too intertwined unfortunately, that when you eat lots of carbohydrates, insulin "spikes," and, after many years of repeated insulin spiking, this leads to insulin resistance, worn out pancreatic beta cells, or both.

Search high and low, near and far, up and down, and over and out… But you're unlikely to find much of anything that is very convincing that suggests that any part of this story is true. If you do manage to find a little fragment of something somewhere, it is usually not relevant to real life, and real life has an avalanche of contradictions against any theories one could build up to validate this myth somehow.

To begin with, as we touched upon in the chapter on Glycogen, those who are insulin sensitive typically have a good "spike" in insulin when they eat food. This allows glucose to quickly be packed away into muscle cells for later use and both the blood glucose levels and the insulin levels to return to baseline (and in a really insulin sensitive person like myself, blood glucose levels hardly ever rise – even after a big meal with hundreds of grams of carbohydrates).

This appears to be the healthy response to eating. Insulin resistant people have a totally different response, producing hardly any "spike" in insulin at all, followed by insulin levels gradually travelling up and then kind of lingering up high for a while before coming back down again. These peculiarities already gray the definitive lines that most people sketch up in their minds after reading through the popular Paleo materials.

More important are the obvious examples. Take a look globally. Are there correlations between the consumption of a diet heavily weighted towards carbohydrates and insulin resistance? Well, there is a relationship. It's one called an "inverse correlation." That's one a them correlations that are like, reverse. In other words, the higher the diet is in carbohydrates by percentage of calories, the lower the likelihood for insulin resistance and things that often result from insulin resistance (such as obesity, early puberty, nearsightedness, type 2 diabetes, PCOS, and many others).

Although you shouldn't need much more than a trip to Africa or Asia to really convince you that carbohydrates, the staples of a few billion people living in those areas, are inherently fattening compared to say, the diet of the Pima Indians (one of the highest fat diets in the world). I have found some of the research coming out of Africa to be particularly interesting. This includes the pioneering work of people like T.L. "Peter" Cleave, Hugh Trowell, and Denis Burkitt.

T.L. Cleave had the opportunity to witness the health outcomes of what could very well be the world's highest carbohydrate diet…

"90 per cent of the calorific intake in the rural Zulu is provided by carbohydrates…"

Yet the rural Zulu were free from what Cleave coined "the Saccharine Disease," which included…

"Dental decay and pyorrhea; gastric and duodenal ulcer and other forms of indigestion; obesity, diabetes, and coronary disease; constipation, with its complications of varicose veins and hemorrhoids; and primary Escherichia coli infections, like appendicitis, cholecystitis (with or without gall-stones), and primary infections of the urinary tract. The same applies to certain skin conditions."

Denis Burkitt made similar observations in Uganda and other parts of Africa, where dietary composition was typically 70-80% of dietary calories as carbohydrates, if not more depending on the area and time of year.

Of course, none of this should be all that shocking. After all, we are primates. Most primates are highly frugivorous (they eat fruit-based diets), and consume 70-90% of their dietary calories as carbohydrates as a general rule – although of course there are a few species that are exceptions to this. I'm sure, out in the jungle, obesity runs rampant amongst these cousins of ours! Too bad they haven't evolved enough to read Gary Taubes's *Good Calories, Bad Calories*[3]. I guess diabetes and obesity is the consequence of their failure to evolve more intelligent brains. Fruit must make you stupid too.

And I hate to bring this up, as there are a lot of other factors involved in this (protein restriction allows one to eat far more calories without weight gain), and these guys are

---

[3] Taubes actually bases much of his argument against refined carbohydrates using T.L. Cleave's logic, who he cites repeatedly throughout the book. And then goes on to blame all carbohydrates, even though Cleave's research, and pretty much all research ever done, shows the protective effect of unrefined carbohydrates against things like obesity, insulin resistance, and hyperglycemia/diabetes. Cherry farmers in Washington have been trying to recruit Taubes for picking season for years. He's like the Lebron James of the industry.

completely bananas, but the fruit-based, low-fat raw vegans can certainly put away incredible amounts of carbohydrates and still have body fat levels of a concentration camp victim (as they love to point out to the Paleo crowd). Last week I watched one video of a kid who lost 140 pounds eating 750 grams of sugar per day, for example (a year later I co-authored a book with him actually – *The Vegan Solution: Why the Vegan Diet Often Fails and How to Fix It*). But it's not just them. Almost anyone can eat a fruit-based diet and lose tremendous amounts of body fat – even if calorie intake is very high. I had one guy lose over 50 pounds eating as much fruit as he could before noon every day last year – a guy that is extremely insulin resistant in fact.

Speaking of insulin resistance and carbohydrates, why is it that every book about reversing type 2 Diabetes is about increasing carbohydrate intake and eating tons of unrefined carbohydrates? I'm talking about the likes of John McDougall, Neal Barnard, Joel Fuhrman, Julian Whitaker, and Doug Graham here. I read quite a bit of material from all of these authors during my research for *180 Degree Diabetes*. Joel Fuhrman claims to have tremendous success with diabetes reversal and makes some great comments on the "carbs raise insulin" myth...

"So, it is certainly true – as the advocates of animal-food-rich diets, such as Atkins, Heller, Sears, and others proclaim – carbohydrates drive up insulin levels temporarily. These writers, however, have not presented the data in accurate fashion. A diet revolving around unrefined carbohydrates (fruits, vegetables, whole grains, and legumes) will not raise blood sugars or insulin levels. Studies have shown that such a diet can reduce fasting insulin levels 30-40 percent in just three weeks."

And his results are impressive, even if he is exaggerating the truth here a little bit...

"More than 90 percent of my Type II diabetics are able to eventually discontinue their insulin within the first month. "

But it should really be no surprise, as the study of high-carbohydrate, high-fiber diets – known in scientific study as the ol' HCF diet, has always yielded good results with type 2 diabetics.

High-carbohydrate, high-fiber diets for insulin-treated men with diabetes mellitus

JW Anderson and K Ward

The effects of high-carbohydrate, high plant fiber (HCF) diets on glucose and lipid metabolism of 20 lean men receiving insulin therapy for diabetes mellitus were evaluated on a metabolic ward. All men received control diets for an average of 7 days followed by HCF diets for an average of 16 days. Diets were designed to be weight-maintaining and there were no significant alterations in body weight. The daily dose of insulin was lower for each patient on the HCF diet than on the control diet. The average insulin dose was reduced from 26 +/- 3 units/day (mean +/- SEM) on the control diets to 11 +/- 3 (P less than 0.001) on the HCF diets. On the HCF diets, insulin therapy could be discontinued in nine patients receiving 15 to 20 units/day and in two patients receiving 32 units/day. Fasting and 3-hr postprandial plasma glucose values were lower in most patients on the HCF diets than on the control diets despite lower insulin doses. Serum cholesterol values dropped from 206 +/- 10 mg/dl on the control diets to 147 +/- 5 (P less than 0.001) on the HCF diet; average fasting serum triglyceride values were not significantly altered on the HCF diets. These studies suggest that HCF diets may be the dietary therapy of choice for certain patients with the maturity-onset type of diabetes.

http://www.ajcn.org/content/32/11/2312

Now let's not get too carried away. I could easily write a book bashing the myopic views of those that think plant-based vegetarian diets are fabulous when it comes not only to health, but even the control and/or reversal of type 2 diabetes. Only someone who can have a normal insulin and glucose response to a few slices of really good New York pizza and a big ass Sprite can consider themselves "cured" of the condition of diabetes. And carbohydrate restriction as well as fat restriction both cause the glucose and insulin response to pizza to get WORSE. I have devised strategies that actually improve the glucose and insulin response to common triggers of hyperglycemia, and that have no rebound effect.

Once again, what helps in the short-term usually hurts in the long-term, because short-term changes triggered by nutrition are often the mirror opposite of the long-term consequences. Just like with cutting calories to lose weight. Yeah, it makes you lose weight and all of your blood lipids and glucose levels and insulin levels and sensitivity and ALL of that improves. But it ignores the fact that decreasing caloric intake decreases metabolism and increases appetite and stress hormone production – leading to a huge rebound effect and a long-term worsening in all categories. The same could be said for all of these shitty diets that remove entire food groups. Keep your carbs or fats low enough for long enough, and eating even small amounts of the stuff you've been restricting will cause your blood sugar and insulin to go into the stratosphere (at least until you've eaten WITHOUT such restrictions for an extended period of time).

My best assessment of the physiology going on with insulin resistance and elevated insulin levels, although I have no plans of going into this in excruciating detail, is completely different than the carbs raise glucose raises insulin fairy tale circulating in the Paleo world.

For starters, as we will get into in the next chapter, carbohydrates do not raise glucose or insulin levels. I encourage people to add carbohydrates to their diets to lower glucose and insulin levels, and they typically have fantastic results with it.

This is probably due to the fact that carbohydrates, particularly high-glycemic starches like grains and potatoes, decrease glucocorticoids – like cortisol. The lower the cortisol level, the greater the insulin sensitivity – barring adrenal failure/fatigue. Thus, glucose gets cleared easily from the bloodstream into the cells for storage and immediate use – like it does in a healthy person. When insulin resistance decreases, basal insulin levels naturally fall. When glucocorticoid secretion is reduced, you also see less overall activity in the adrenal glands. The adrenal hormones RAISE blood sugar, whereas insulin lowers blood sugar. Turn down glucocorticoid secretion – and carbohydrates play a vital role in achieving that, and both glucose and insulin levels fall. Neato.

Excesses of cortisol are known to cause not only impairment to glucose metabolism and full-blown type 2 diabetes, but basically every complication that comes with it – including belly fat, moon face (sometimes called "carbo face" by some of the weaker-minded people in the Paleo community), macular degeneration, reduced peripheral circulation, immune system impairment, increased risk of heart disease – you name it.

Perhaps the most interesting component is that the sex hormones like testosterone and progesterone, as well as thyroid (which controls the rate at which those hormones are synthesized), oppose the glucocorticoids. With aging, you see a steady rise of glucocorticoids and a steady fall of thyroid and sex hormones. And with that you get steadily worsening body composition, health, and the accompanying rises in glucose and insulin levels (note: all this while eating LESS total food and FEWER carbohydrates).

Anyway, I could go on endless tangents here. But you should at least have recognized the greater complexity behind human metabolism than some stupid theory about carbohydrates causing a chronic elevation in insulin and glucose levels because of what happens in the hour that follows ingesting food. What happens in an hour after eating is pretty irrelevant in the grand scheme of things, especially over decades and generations.

Spiking insulin and glucose levels actually looks like it protects against insulin resistance, and can even reverse insulin resistance. This is all reminiscent of the good ol' days when they thought that using your heart would cause it to wear out faster. Turns out that really stressing out your heart with some exercise just made the whole circulatory system stronger, and your heart go longer. I believe the same could be said with our glucose metabolism. You don't develop superhuman glucose metabolism by avoiding carbs just like you don't win races by sitting on the couch.

More on this in the next chapter, as we look at what could very well be the world's most impressive documented case of insulin resistance reversal – and it happened not despite, but in part BECAUSE 250 grams of carbohydrates were added per day.

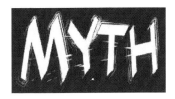

Low-carb Diets Ensure Low Glucose and Insulin Levels

"It is of interest that diets high in fibre-rich cereals and tuberous vegetables tend to result in an improvement in basal blood glucoses."
~Denis Burkitt, Hugh Trowell, and Kenneth Heaton. *Dietary Fibre, Fibre-Depleted Foods and Disease*

I often mention this quote because it is simple, straightforward, and true. But those under the influence of Paleo often have their heads explode when they read it. That's a good thing. Believing in some simple and tidy theory about how carbs raise insulin and blood sugar and cause insulin resistance and diabetes is absurd. The sooner you can get smarter the better. This glycemic index stuff has really thrown people's heads out into left field, because people have become obsessed with what happens in the hour after eating, which is meaningless in terms of the long-term portrait of obesity, diabetes, and related disorders.

From an article I released in June of 2011…

It is a common belief that starch, or any type of carbohydrate – particularly high-glycemic starches like potatoes, raises insulin. In the low-carb circles you see the idea floating around that carbohydrate ingestion raises glucose, which in turn raises insulin. Insulin increases fat storage, therefore carbohydrates make you fat and are the cause of the obesity epidemic.

Gross oversimplifications that the human mind can easily grasp are always popular – regardless of what the oversimplifications are intended to explain. In the health sphere, they are prevalent. The carbs = insulin = fat myth is one of the greatest and most easily refutable. It's up there with the great fat = cholesterol = clogged arteries = heart attack theory that is simple, easy to follow, makes sense to those who don't study it, and is completely silly and a total misrepresentation of the etiology of heart disease.

As always, it depends on context. In my program designed to, among other things, restore insulin sensitivity, I do not say "eat starch and you will live happily ever after."

Instead, I say something like… "Eat plenty of food, don't overexert yourself physically or mentally, get plenty of sleep, eat only saturated fats and keep omega 6 polyunsaturated fat ingestion pretty low, get sufficient but not excessive amounts of quality protein, have plenty of salt, and eat plenty of high-glycemic starch at every meal. And something sweet too, sometimes a lot."

This generally lowers the activity of the sympathetic nervous system, increases thyroid activity, improves glycogen storage, and starts shuttling glucose from ingested food into muscle cells where it creates muscle growth and the generation of heat and energy. This reduces insulin resistance. If you are insulin resistant and have high fasting insulin levels as a result of this insulin resistance, then insulin levels will fall dramatically on this program. For example, below is an email sent to me by someone who has followed 180DegreeHealth for over a year.

A traumatic childhood stress caused this person to suddenly become insulin resistant (as chronic stress hormone secretion is the primary root cause of insulin resistance) and gain something like 60 pounds in a year if I recall correctly from our email exchanges. She has had blood sugar regulation and thyroid problems ever since, which she tried to medicate with a low-carbohydrate diet to varying degrees of restriction.

She has spent the last 4 years on a low-carbohydrate diet, and her fasting insulin levels have varied between a VERY high 14 and 33 IU/m. But after just four months of loosely following my program to increase metabolism with special attention to eating high-starch and low-PUFA (polyunsaturated fats), her insulin has fallen all the way down to a perfect 4.7 IU/m. Her fasting glucose has fallen nearly in half to a level that probably scared the doc into thinking (mistakenly) that she was about to fall into a hypoglycemic coma (yet she no longer experiences high-adrenaline states that many call 'hypoglycemia' like she did on a carbohydrate-restricted diet).

If I am not mistaken she did not lose a single pound of body weight during this time, so any drop in insulin cannot be attributed to temporary weight loss or calorie restriction. Her calorie intake has not dropped at all, but presumably increased as she was instructed to intentionally eat beyond appetite. Following the next two very important sentences is the email she sent me.

If you are still under the influence of low-carb dogma, and believe that eating carbohydrates will raise your insulin levels, snap out of it. In the right context, carbs are your best metabolic friend, and what passes as science and physiology in the low-carb realm is a complete scientific sasquatch...

"Just got some labs back and thought I'd share them with you.

I am still low in iron, which is surprising to me considering I eat red meat, but I think the high RT3 and celiac disease all play a part in this.

On the other hand I am quite pleased with my blood sugars and insulin levels.

For reference here are my PRIOR glucose and insulin labs:
<u>October 2009</u>:

Glucose: 90 (60-110)
Insulin: 17.9 (3-22)

<u>March 2010</u>:

Glucose: 87 (60-110)
Insulin: 14.6 (3-22)

<u>May 2010</u>:

Glucose random sampling: 97 (50-140)

<u>August 2010</u>:

Glucose: 95 (60-110)
Insulin: 33 (3-22)

<u>December 2010</u>:

Glucose random sampling: 94 (50-140)

<u>May 2011</u> *(Four months of eating a high starch low PUFA diet – about 250 carbs daily)*

Glucose: 49 (65-100) *
Adiponectin: 2.3 (>2.7)

Insulin: 4.7 (functional range <5.4 IU/m; normal lab range 3-22)
Pro-insulin: <5 (<42)
HBA1C: 5.9 (4-6)**
HOMA-IR: 0.6 (<2.8) ***
C-Peptide: 1.9 (<2.2)

*I have no idea why my glucose is so low. I did not feel even slightly hypoglycaemic. I generally feel fantastic in terms of hunger and cravings so am slightly puzzled. Still, if the test was performed using a normal lab range of 50-110; I would only be slightly under it. Still, I think a FBG of 49 is a HECK of a lot better than a FBG of 97!

**Not quite sure why my HBA1C isn't in the optimal <5.4 range if glucose and insulin are so excellent. HBA1C is an average of blood sugars over a three month period though, so the HBA1C may be lagging behind in terms of including blood sugars from the first few months of [rest and refeeding] when my blood sugars were a lot higher than they are now.

*** My previous HOMA-IR was 4.1. HOMA-IR is a marker of insulin resistance and diabetes risk, so I was clearly extremely insulin resistant and now appear to have an extremely LOW level of insulin resistance.

When the person who wrote this caught wind of the fact that I was putting this book out, she was eager to give me another update 9 months after she sent me this original email. In her most recent email, you can see what I'm talking about when I say that in a healthy person glucose levels should be pretty stable and consistent all day – even after eating high-glycemic starches alleged to cause "wild blood sugar swings and insulin resistance" according to the leading authorities in the Paleo and low-carb world.

She writes:

"Hi Matt,

How are you? Have I missed the deadline for the book? Or can I add something to it? I thought you might be interested in my numbers a year into a high carb diet... I got my fasting and post meal glucose numbers done sporadically. Here is the breakdown:

Monday fasting a.m.: 84

Monday two hours after lunch: 84

Tuesday two hours after breakfast: 84

Wednesday fasting a.m.: 79

Wednesday three hours after breakfast: 75

Clearly, my insulin sensitivity is fully restored. I no longer get hypos, cravings or hunger. I eat three well balanced meals a day and feel good. It is also important to note to the carb phobics that I have not gained any weight by switching to a high carb diet."

We are now working together to complete the repair of her teeth after they "fell apart" during her years on a low-carb diet. She has noted great improvement since switching to a more starch-based diet. She was pretty surprised I imagine, as was I, when her dental health spiraled down not eating any refined sugar or starches at all. It seems that refined sugar and carbohydrates simply must be the culprit at first glance, but adding white flour and white sugar to people's diets who have incurred tooth problems on a low-carb diet, and seeing drastic improvement in dental health, has proven to me that it has a lot more to do with what's going on in the inside, and the health of a person as a whole. No shortage of surprises when you're exploring human health, that's for sure!

I am totally serious when I say that I know of no more complete and thorough documented reversal of insulin resistance ever achieved through diet and lifestyle manipulation. Going from 4.1 to 0.6 on a HOMA Insulin Resistance test is absolutely phenomenal. 1.0 is considered perfect – from what I understand 1.0 is the established baseline from testing many insulin sensitive young men. And, if all my audience members were monitoring such physiological changes, I'm sure you would see that this would be the common response – not a fluke or an exception. As I mentioned in a previous chapter, just last week I was contacted by a type 2 diabetic that has already seen her postmeal glucose levels go from 359 to 132 mg/dl in less than 3 weeks. I witnessed the same changes myself as I diligently tracked my blood glucose levels from starting fasting levels in the 90's to a consistent fasting level below 70 mg/dl. This also included 1-hour postmeal levels as low as 75 mg/dl even after large, mixed meals with as much as 2 large baked potatoes – this just 4 weeks after seeing a postmeal glucose spike to 173 mg/dl coming off one of those stupid starvation diets recommended for overcoming diabetes.

You will often see long-term low-carbers having abysmal glucose and insulin levels. You can run from carbs, but you can't hide. There is only a sugar packet or so worth of glucose in your entire bloodstream at any given time. It doesn't take much glucose to be liberated from muscle or liver glycogen or to be created from the breakdown of ingested protein to create high levels of glucose in the blood. Low-carb diets cause the adrenal glands to crank, and as long as they are cranking, they are working hard to drive blood glucose levels UP. Fasting glucose in the 90's or higher is typical of a low-carber, even one that went into the diet perfectly insulin sensitive with rock bottom fasting glucose levels. And eating something as insignificant as a half of a sweet potato can drive blood sugar levels up to all-time highs.

It is common knowledge that avoiding carbohydrates makes returning to eating them a nightmare at first, with wilder blood sugar swings, more gas and bloating, more pimples and cravings, fat gain…

But only through persistence and fixing the core of glucose dysregulation can we return to eating carbs and having them affect us favorably. The sooner you start the better. Because glucose, as you will later read, is the ultimate source of cellular energy. Accept no substitutes.

The diabetes and insulin resistance scare is scary indeed. And, when looking through a very narrow perspective, I fully understand that carbohydrates appear to be the villain. I mean hey, here we are with a long list of disorders that can be traced back to high levels of glucose in the bloodstream. And carbs are like pure glucose man! It's a government conspiracy that tells us to eat 6-11 servings of grains per day! And what about the Eskimos derpie, derp!! Pemmican man! Pemmican!!![4]

Yeah I went through that phase too. Nothing to be ashamed about. But there's simply more to the story. More than I ever could have imagined when I first attempted to take on the field of health and nutrition. The more you learn the less you know about this mysterious human organism. I promise you that! And I can promise you that there is no magical macronutrient ratio or dietary prescription that is gonna save humanity from all its perils! So, per the advice of Dave Coulier… "Cut it out!"

---

[4] I don't have any hard data to support this hypothesis, but I think there is probably a tight correlation between the degree in which something feels like it makes sense and is correct and the degree in which it is wrong. In other words, the more you think something is right, and the more sense it makes, the more wrong you are about it!

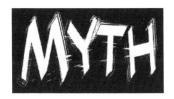

Lack of Genetic Adaptation to Modern Foods Causes Food Sensitivities

I kinda dropped some hints about my stance on this earlier in the book. And in terms of how a person's life is influenced by their dietary beliefs, this ends up being about as important as it gets.

In the Paleo world, you see grains forbidden, dairy discouraged unless the quality is impeccable and "well tolerated," and now, thanks to the success of Robb Wolf and his tendency to err on the safe side, the recommendation to remove all legumes and nightshade vegetables from the diet as well. Because of this hyperawareness about food sensitivities, there is plenty more encouragement given to people about pinpointing other foods that they are sensitive to and removing those as well.

And it's true. Foods have all kinds of chemicals in them that can elicit a reaction. Salicylates, oxalates, lectins… we could go on to list dozens of potential allergens.

And yes, there is certainly a time and place for removing things that people react to. These inflammatory reactions trigger an immune response and subsequent release of inflammatory cytokines, cortisol, SOCS-3 (thought to promote obesity), and other harmful byproducts. This, I agree, is bad. But I'm disheartened by all this dietary restriction because it is just a temporary bandaid for a much larger root problem – an overly reactive inflammatory system. And dietary restriction, if taken too far, becomes a neurotic prison. Meanwhile, long-term, I've rarely if ever seen anyone restrict their way to health – walling themselves off from society and consuming only their handful of "safe" foods.

Immune system regulation is a very complex system that I personally don't fully understand. I don't think anyone does. All we have is a pile of clues pointing us towards the root cause. One thing is for certain, basically all inflammatory conditions are on the rise worldwide. Autoimmune disease, autism, asthma, food allergies, and the most common degenerative diseases like heart disease (all of which are known to be caused primarily by inflammation), are all increasing. The question is, "why?"

Is it because of dairy and grains? Well, considering that we are eating less of them than in the past, this is doubtful. While we also hear about changes in wheat and dairy products to contain more gluten and a different type of casein, this still seems far-fetched. It shouldn't be causing, for example, increased allergies to nuts, eggs, pet dander, or pollen. It shouldn't be causing sensitivity to various chemicals found in common household products and the like.

The bottom line is that we do not know exactly what is causing the big increase in inflammation. But there is no question that there is an epidemic of inflammation, and that inflammation is the primary concern that we face, collectively, as a society in terms of our health. But there are clues and theories that seem certain to be at least part of the picture.

Before we get to those, I will say that while a Paleo diet can, and has helped to relieve many people in the short-term by removing many potential triggers of inflammation, one thing that I absolutely haven't seen from the diet is an extinguishing of the inflammatory tendency in the first place. There is, to be perfectly clear, a big difference between a cause of inflammation and a trigger of inflammation. I don't see people reducing their allergies, only increasing them – as a general rule. And avoiding an allergen is not conquering the hyperinflammatory state that lies at the root of all overly-inflammatory reactions. I wish I had a nickel for every person that has found a highly-restricted diet – particularly Paleo and low-carb, to actually increase or create higher levels of sensitivity – especially to food.

In fact, in the Paleo world, it's almost seen as a rite of passage that you remove gluten from your diet long enough to have a severe reaction to it when you put it back into the diet. This self-fulfilling prophecy strikes me as very eerie. Most people don't have a negative reaction to gluten, but put them on a Paleo diet for long enough and they might develop one. Paleo enthusiasts use this as great evidence of the evil, villainous ways of El Gluten. That scum sucking pig! That son of a motherless goat!

But because I see people become hypersensitive to a lot more than just wheat products during their Paleo stints – like my ex-girlfriend who developed deadly shellfish allergies suddenly while restricting carbohydrates, I can't help but raise some red flags about it. I strongly suspect that Paleo has a remarkable ability to create food allergies and sensitivities.

I believe it does this for two primary reasons, which I think are the two primary reasons for the rise in inflammation that we've seen on a global scale over the past century...

1) Overconsumption of linoleic acid and arachidonic acid
2) Decreased metabolic rate

The first item in the list may sound like something you have never heard about before, but you have – it just came packaged differently. If you have heard of omega 3 fatty acids or the many wondrous benefits of fish oil, you have certainly heard about the connection between the type of fat we eat and inflammation. Omega 3 fat is considered to basically be the opposite of linoleic and arachidonic acids. While LA and AA generally promote inflammatory processes, omega 3 counteracts it. There is greater complexity there, as with most things, but that is generally true.

But the gist of it all is that we have a network of eicosanoid molecules involved in the regulation of many functions. We have tiny molecules that cause bronchoconstriction, we have tiny molecules that cause bronchodilation. What's interesting is that the balance between constriction and dilation (of the lungs, of blood vessels, and so forth), or whether we produce more pro-inflammatory or anti-inflammatory molecules, is the fatty acid balance of our diets.

So if we look at molecules like some of the interleukins or thromboxanes, some of the most powerful pro-inflammatory molecules, we see that the relative balance of these two basic types of fat determines how much of this inflammatory stuff that we produce. It really does appear to be pretty straightforward like this. If the cells are loaded up with lots of AA, the body will produce more inflammation in response to anything that triggers inflammation. This could be any kind of food. It could be an infection. It could be injury, a bee sting, you name it. Inflammatory molecules are always going to be there in any kind of inflammatory situation, but the degree of that inflammatory reaction is highly dependent on the fatty acid balance of our cells.

And modern human cells are frickin' loaded with tons of LA and AA, the generally pro-inflammatory fats! Yes, we can actually see that in our tissues and even the breast milk of nursing moms like we talked about, that the composition of the diet in terms of fatty acid intake has a huge bearing on the balances of fatty acids in the body. In turn, these fatty acid balances determine the degree in which we produce inflammation in response to potential triggers.

Interestingly, the biggest dietary change of the 20th century was not the brand new incorporation of wheat and dairy products into the diet. Far from it. The question we should be asking ourselves is "what did change?" Well, a lot. We certainly eat more refined grains than we used to, including refined sugar, refined flour, and other refined grains. But many societies seem to be doing alright for themselves on refined grains. White rice, for example, usually proves itself to be protective against most modern disease any time it is studied.

The biggest dietary change by far was the shift towards the consumption of large amounts of vegetable and seed oils. Prior to the 20th century, we lacked the technology to turn something like corn into an oil. But the 20th century made this possible, and so we rapidly replaced all of our oils and butter and lard and tallow with vegetable-based versions. Soy and corn oil quickly became the most consumed oils in diets all over the world, particularly in the United States where this stuff grows like there's no tomorrow.

These oils are the most concentrated sources of linoleic acid (LA). LA is a precursor molecule to the formation of inflammatory molecules that increase clotting, bronchoconstriction, vasoconstriction, and other things clearly linked to the allergic process as well as many degenerative diseases (increased vasoconstriction being something associated with hypertension and heart disease, as is an increased tendency to form deadly blood clots in heart attacks and strokes).

Perhaps just as important was the fact that we started feeding livestock with soy, corn, and the like at around the same time. While the fat composition of ruminant animals like sheep and cows aren't significantly impacted by the fatty acids in their diet, pork and poultry, like humans, have pretty much a linear relationship between the fats they eat and the fat they wear.

Thus, pork fat and organ meats as well as eggs and poultry, are the richest sources of Arachidonic Acid (AA), discovered to be an even more potent pro-inflammatory fatty acid as mentioned in this Floyd Chilton quote used earlier in the book…

"Research has proven that a high AA diet has the potential actually to change normal immune responses to abnormal, exaggerated ones. A study carried out in 1997 by Dr. Darshan S. Kelley and colleagues at the Western Human Nutrition Research Center in California showed that people on high-AA diets generated four times as many inflammatory cells after a flu vaccination as people on low-AA diets."

Hey man, even feeding lots of seed oil to salmon makes them an inflammatory food!

"In humans, eating lots of LA isn't such a big deal, because, as we discussed, we aren't good at turning LA into AA. But because the salmon are so very good at moving those fatty acids through those conversions, when salmon eat a lot of LA, a great deal of AA ends up in that last bucket. And of course, when we eat that AA-loaded salmon, we end up with lots of AA in our own buckets."

This has obvious implications in the rise of adverse reactions to certain foods and substances in our environments. It does a great deal to explain why we are seeing big rises in inflammation, whereas foods that were introduced to the human diet 10,000 or more years ago absolutely does not.

I am left saying, fairly confidently, that if a person has a hypersensitive or overinflammatory reaction to any food, whether that be post-agricultural food or pre-agricultural food, it is because of THE PERSON, not the food. People love to blame their problems on particular evil foods, when it is usually the person's poor response to the food that is to blame – stemming back to the perversion in their inflammatory response from factors totally unrelated to what cavemen did or didn't eat. And then, of course, this often leads to some huge conquest to warn every human on earth that "x" food is the root of all evil. Sigh.

Factor #2, I suspect, is decreased metabolic rate (which may also be related to these fatty acids). We know that metabolic rate is in decline. Even the New York Times put out an article called "Rethinking 98.6" because that temperature has ceased to become "normal." Inflammation has a distinct pro-stress, anti-metabolic property, but the linoleic acid in vegetable oil seems uniquely capable of causing a reduction in metabolic rate through all kinds of mechanisms – mechanisms too complex to fully dive into here.

Regardless of the root cause of the collective decline in metabolism (I could easily put together an equally compelling argument pinning the decline on the rising popularity of dieting instead of these pro-inflammatory fatty acids), I have some reason to suspect that it is involved with the perversion of the inflammatory response. It is more of a hunch than anything, as I have watched, for example, the development of autoimmune disease come and go based entirely on metabolic rate. You also see those that have undergone weight loss surgery, and thus obliterating their metabolic rate, developing autoimmune disease and other inflammatory conditions at an increased rate.

Same goes for hard-training athletes, particularly women who are more susceptible.

A more direct example with obsessive food prison comes from a girl who once blogged at great length about the wide variety of allergens and triggers in various foods. The blog was called Plant Poisons and Rotten Stuff and featured the trials and tribulations of a sick and hypersensitive girl that had negative reactions to damn near everything and was forced to eat a diet known as The Failsafe Diet for the hyperallergenic mofos of the universe.

It was a rough place to be. A refuge for some truly crippled people that were all but completely owned by their diets. Then one day, she got thyroid meds. Problem solved. And the blog basically came to a sudden and abrupt halt.

I can't exactly say what the anti-inflammatory effects of increasing thyroid hormone are. And to be honest, I've grown somewhat tired of trying to speculate as to the physiological basis of what can plainly be observed and witnessed with two eyes. People often overcome or improve upon inflammatory conditions, including overcoming food sensitivities, when raising metabolic rate.

The bottom line is that, with my personal experience and research into the matter, I simply can't support the idea that there is something inherently wrong about grains, dairy, and other agricultural era foods for our species. It is a myth. And it's also unrealistic to think that, as a society, we are going to depart from the consumption of such foods. Because damn, grains and dairy make for some good eats. And as far as I'm concerned, both can play an important role in increasing metabolic rate and in turn decreasing inflammation.

As a final note, there is one thing that I never really considered until I had written this book. It seems so obvious and simple and could very well be why so many, like myself, experience…

A huge decrease in inflammatory conditions on a Paleo type of diet

Followed by a huge increase in inflammatory conditions 3-12 months later

Ever have some really nasty inflammatory condition? What did you do? You went and had some cortisone injected in there didn't ya? That's right, our most potent anti-allergy, anti-autoimmunity, anti-inflammation substance.

I think what may very well be happening is that during the early stages of adopting the diet – the honeymoon period, cortisol secretion is much higher. This wipes out all inflammation. But over time, depending on the adrenal fortitude of the person playing around with the diet, the adrenal glands finally wear out and start producing LESS than ideal levels of cortisol. Thus, the frequently-observed swing from less inflammation, more energy, and fat loss to more inflammation, less energy, and fat gain.

Think about that as you read through some of the Paleo stories at the end of the book.

Burning Fat as Fuel is Superior

Perhaps you have to be an extreme exerciser to feel this, but no one who does a large amount of exercise or trains hard would ever pick fat over glucose as a primary fuel source. For a while, I was thrown off of this. When I started eating a fat-based diet I noticed that I never ran out of gas. I could go hiking all day and...

1) Not get hungry
2) Never feel a dip in energy
3) Not even feel tired at the end of the day

I mistook all of these changes for signs of superior athletic performance and endurance. Hey man! This fat really is the ultimate fuel source!

Of course, when you are out doing a lot of hiking, you don't really know how fast you are going. It wasn't until I went hiking with other people that I realized that I couldn't keep up. You bet I could hike all day long without even getting tired. But I didn't realize how slow I was going compared to my usual pace, which was previously much faster than my hiking partners, but now much slower. Even an out-of-shape fish biologist with a potbelly that I went out hiking with left me in the dust. I had a full-on set of 6-pack abs, but just couldn't find that higher gear that I used to have when eating carby stuff all day.

This is all because fat is low-octane fuel. When you burn fat for fuel effectively, you basically have an unlimited supply. You can burn thousands of calories and never get really fatigued. You just keep on truckin'. This is often misperceived as an improvement in performance, but it ain't.

Rather, our glucose reserves are smaller than our fat reserves. So if you burn glucose, you need to fill the tank more often. If you exercise hard, you need to eat often, and feel hungry as hell all day long. This is not a bad thing. This is just how it goes. Ferrari engines burn a lot of gas and have small tanks. I'm sorry.

If you don't believe that carbohydrates are superior for exercise performance, you might also hop on a piece of cardio-type of equipment at a gym and see how many calories you can burn in a 20-minute session on fat vs. glucose. You'll see pretty quickly that you can perform at a much higher level if your glycogen reserves are full going into it after a big carbohydrate feast the day before – or sometimes even a few hours or even minutes before.

Granted, as we talked about in the chapter on glycogen, getting glycogen reserves maxed out isn't simply a matter of eating as many carbohydrates as you can. So I'm not bashing the other macronutrients here or even saying that someone on a Paleo diet couldn't achieve fantastic athletic performance. I think it's possible. Just picking on the simple fallacy that fat oxidation or running on ketones is a superior thing to glucose oxidation. It is not. Plain and simple.

There's really no secret here. If you want to perform at a higher level athletically, and recuperate more quickly, the higher your carbohydrate consumption the better. That's why 99% of competitive athletes get more of their dietary calories from carbohydrates than they do from fats. They would likely eat maggots and drink turpentine if it made them perform better. They don't do it for health but for performance. So the question remains, even if glucose is the best fuel for exercise, is it healthier to be burning it for energy?

I think the answer to this is another clear "yes." One of the main differences between young people and old people is that old people burn more fat and less glucose for their energy supply – just as we see that insulin resistant people get more of their energy supply from fat than they do from glucose. These are not positives, but serious negatives. You'll also see similar things arising with cancer. One of the hallmarks of cancer is burning fat for fuel instead of glucose, and a departure away from a glycolytic metabolism.

What you really want to see in a healthy person is a very active oxidative metabolism that burns glucose up like an inferno to produce ATP. This is a hallmark of being in a healthy metabolic state.

Things that reinforce the burning of fat vs. the burning of glucose would be things that increase the reliance upon fat for fuel. Those things would be…

1) Low heart rate endurance exercise
2) Sedentarism
3) Excessive fat intake
4) Stress
5) Not using your brain actively (watching television, doing mundane tasks)

Plain and simple, most everything points to being physically active – particularly glucose-using activities like interval and resistance training, using your mind actively and creatively to learn and solve problems, and eating a buttload of carbs for health, longevity, and even keeping insulin and blood glucose levels low. Don't be a fat phobe, but get plenty of carbohydrates – enough to keep glycogen full and always have access to as much glucose as your body cares to burn.

High Protein Diets Raise Your Metabolism

"It has been clearly established that a high protein diet lowers the metabolic rate, [therefore] symptoms of hypothyroidism will be aggravated... Hypoglycemia may be controlled on the high protein diet, but the other symptoms of thyroid deficiency which usually accompany hypoglycemia are aggravated."
~Broda Barnes

"For all the hoopla around the high-protein diet craze, the gurus of this movement had one thing right: Protein is much more effective at filling you up than either carbohydrates or fat. Thus, you tend to eat less at individual meals, supporting quicker weight loss in the short term.

However, this form of eating has minimal impact on longer-term signals. Eventually – over the course of weeks or months – you're driven to take in more calories – or spend fewer calories..."
~Linda Bacon

The word "metabolism" has been molested like the girl with the dragon tattoo. Abominations like "exercise raises metabolism" are spread based on the belief that burning off some calories therefore means your metabolism is increased. Hogwash. When I think of metabolism, I think of basal metabolic rate, or BMR. That is how much energy your body produces AT REST. Endurance exercise will make your BMR plummet to next to nothing, as does most exercise. That's one of the reasons hard training athletes have low pulse rates (reduced resting metabolism). But they also tend to have low body temperatures. I have taken my body temperature from a toasty 98 degrees F to 96.2 degrees F with exercise. Some boost to metabolism that was! Burning calories with exercise doesn't increase metabolic rate any more than burning gas changes the fuel efficiency of your car.

Protein has suffered from the same flawed logic. Protein is more expensive to digest than any other macronutrient. In other words, the digestion of it requires more energy to be lost than when, say, fat is ingested. And there is a thermal effect from this expense or caloric loss. So like, protein totally raises your metabolism!

It doesn't. Well, if you don't eat enough of ANY macronutrient it will lower your metabolic rate. So yes, it will raise your metabolic rate if you are coming off of a really low protein diet like the 80-10-10 low-fat raw vegan diet (the creator of the diet, Doug Graham, actually champions the diet on its ability to lower body temperature to as low as 93 degrees F!).

"On a low fat raw vegan diet, a typical athlete will have a resting temperature of around 93 degrees. (S)he can warm up as much as desired, play as intensely as possible; the true fever will likely never be reached. Clear thinking becomes the norm, rather than the exception. Efficient functioning is most readily achieved when body temperatures run healthfully, in the lower 90's."

But protein, in excess, is very anti-metabolic, not pro-metabolic. One of the reasons it reduces metabolic rate is BECAUSE so many calories are wasted digesting it. Another is that it is very satiating, so on a high-protein diet you naturally consume fewer calories. At least, statistically-speaking people consume fewer calories when you hike the protein intake high enough.

But all of this is calorie restriction in disguise, and it comes with a great penalty.

There are also some other concerning things about diets that are very high in protein beyond that which is essential to maintain nitrogen balance while taking in sufficient calories. One is that diets high in muscle meats are rich in a lot of pro-inflammatory, anti-metabolic amino acids that cause more inflammation when consumed in large amounts. This includes methionine, cysteine, and tryptophan – and meats are almost always richer in these type of amino acids than proteins found in plant sources. This might also be a factor in why people often develop new allergies and "itis-es" after long-term Paleo eating. Of course, we've already gone over some of the potential perils of consuming an excess of animal protein in general – taking in too much Arachidonic Acid (AA), especially if you are taking in a lot of pork, poultry, organ meats, and eggs.

Then of course we have the uric acid issue, which is very real. Back when I was under the influence of low-carbism, I told a friend of mine that had had a heart attack to really "get his insulin under control" by tightening up on those killer carbs. Within weeks he had a massive attack of gout. Fail. I appreciate his willing guinea-piggedness though. How do you think I learned all this crap in the first place?

I have had others dramatically reduce their uric acid levels once they've gotten off of a mostly meat-based diet.

In reality, after years of seeing the body temperatures/metabolisms of people after they have followed a diet very high in protein, and guiding them towards much higher body temperatures with a change in diet primarily, it's quite obvious that meat, fish, and other concentrated high-quality proteins are most useful when they play a supporting, not a leading role.

Protein is more for building new tissue. That's great. You need it. Plenty. But you don't want to eat so much that you are burning it as a fuel source. You are much better off getting your fuel from what is much more readily used as fuel – carbohydrates and fat. And, the more calories you eat, the less protein you need to maintain or even build lean tissue. Likewise, the more calories you eat from things like starches, fruits, legumes, and grains – the fewer meats, fish, and dairy proteins you need. When you take in, say, 500 grams of starchy carbohydrates and fruits per day, you're probably going to get close to 80 grams of protein packaged with that. Meat can then become more of a condiment, and when it does, metabolism usually responds favorably.

Anyway, there's no need to beat this to death. If you are on a high-protein diet, you will probably be better off when it comes to inflammation and metabolism if you get more like 10-15% of your calories from protein. Certainly no more than 20%. I'm not advocating a meat-free diet. Be open and flexible. Some people need a substantial portion of meat at least once per day to perform at their best. Others could potentially get by with as little as a few ounces of meat per week. But I certainly don't want anyone thinking that eating a pound or more of meat every day is going to ramp up their metabolic rate. That is only going to happen temporarily when coming off of a vegetarian diet, and eventually will become a liability if kept up for too long.

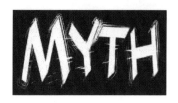

It is Healthy to Lose Weight on a Paleo Diet

"We don't have an obesity (and overweight) epidemic; our epidemic is one of fearmongering and ignorance. Consider the following statements:
Overweight and obesity lead to early death.
Overweight and obesity lead to disease.
We are gaining weight at epidemic rates.
Weight loss improves health and longevity.
You control what you weigh.
Anyone can keep lost weight off if she or he tries hard enough.
Thinner is more attractive.
We can trust the experts to provide accurate information.

For most of us, these statements seem like basic truisms. However, much of what we believe to be true about weight – including all of the statements above – is in fact myth, fueled by the power of money and cultural bias. Public health officials, health advocates, and scientists are complicit (often unintentionally) in supporting and encouraging the lies. The campaign against obesity is not about science or health; its misconceptions about the most basic research are astounding. If you suspend your preconceptions and open yourself to the scientific evidence, a very different picture emerges."

~Linda Bacon; *Health at Every Size*

A lot of people lose weight when they switch to a Paleo diet. Awesome. A lot of people lose weight when they take up meth, or smoking, or get cancer, or go vegan, or do some fasting, or jump on Weight Watchers, or take Phen-Fen or whatever it's called, or go to some Biggest Loser-esque boot camp. So how do we know that it is healthy? Oh, that's right. Because our ancestors ate that way. It's in our DNA. I remember.

I don't think there's a bigger myth on the face of the planet than the weight loss myth. Okay, well, that's a little strong – but it certainly seems to be the biggest and most pervasive myth in the health and fitness industry. The weight loss myth is basically that if you lose body fat, and get lean, it will improve your health. This is a huge rabbit hole, but we will dive into it at least part of the way.

"In America today the medical and public health establishment has managed to transform what has traditionally been considered a vice – physical vanity – into that most sacred of secular virtues: the pursuit of 'health.' In the context of the war on fat it has done so by systematically distorting the available evidence regarding the relationship between weight and health, by severely exaggerating the risks associated with that evidence, and by pretending that an extremely complex subject is actually quite simple.

These are harsh charges, but if anything, they understate the scandal that is the war on fat. Never before in American history has so much junk science been exploited to whip up hysteria about a supposed public health 'epidemic.' The health establishment's constant barrage of scientifically baseless propaganda regarding the relationship between weight and health constitutes nothing less than egregious abuse of the public trust. This propaganda has played a key role in creating a culture that makes tens of

millions of people miserable about their bodies: Worse yet, it has done so for crass economic motives. The war on fat, which is supposedly about making all of us healthy, is really about making some of us rich."
~Paul Campos; *The Obesity Myth*

It's true that carrying around excess body fat is probably not a representation of what could be considered "optimal health." But you should know that, despite our prejudices against it and beliefs that it is causing us all to "drop dead of heart attacks and get diabetes," the actual data that has been gathered suggests that if you are an American citizen over age 65, your greatest mortality and morbidity statistics actually lie in the BMI range of 30-35. Yeah, you read that right. The compiled NHANES data, some of the best data we have on bodyweight and risk factors, actually finds that what is called Stage 1 obesity (BMI 30-35) is protective against degenerative disease and statistically increases the lifespan of an American citizen. You won't see that in the Weight Watchers pamphlet or hear that being talked about on the Biggest Loser.

If you are leaner than that, or heavier than that, you get sick more often and die younger. So much for all this anti-fat hysteria. Being slightly obese isn't exactly as scary as it's made out to be by your favorite diet guru or news network.

So, to begin this conversation, we must acknowledge that having some body fat has been in no way proven to be unhealthy. This same data has shown that if you are physically fit, excess body fat becomes even less of a risk factor and that someone who is "fat AND fit" is much more likely to outlive someone who is thin and unfit.

Likewise, all of the risk factors associated with obesity have shown to be overturnable with some improvements in diet and lifestyle EVEN IF THOSE DIETARY CHANGES DON'T RESULT IN WEIGHT LOSS.

How's your brain doing now? All this suggests, as some of my favorite authors like Linda Bacon, Paul Campos, Laura Fraser, Glenn Gaesser, and Gina Kolata have been shouting for years, that health risks and problems that we normally blame on obesity don't have anything to do with obesity. It's just that many of the diet, lifestyle, socioeconomic, and other conditions that cause increased risk of health problems and early death often cause excess body fat to accumulate as well.

Okay, I'm tired of trying to fit in a ll these quotes in appropriate places. I'm just going to drop them all in one place. I've got nearly 30 pages of great quotes harvested from large stacks of books on this topic. Here is a nice sampling to help you believe that I'm not making this shiz up…

"Despite the fact that there is intense interest now among obesity researchers, physicians, and public health officials in treating obesity as a disease – aggressively – a new view about weight is emerging. This view, which is shared by many eating disorder researchers, nutritionists, exercise physiologists, psychologists, and fat activists, holds that weight is not an accurate measurement of human health – or character.

"The new paradigm about weight acknowledges that dieting is negative and most often doesn't work, and that a more positive approach to health is in order. This view encourages people to stop dieting, to develop lifelong healthy eating and exercise habits instead, and to accept whatever weight they end up with. Some people may shed a few pounds by eating better and exercising more, and others won't; whatever the result, there's nothing more anyone can realistically do about their size."
~Laura Fraser; *Losing It*
"Extensive evidence documents that attempts at dieting typically result in weight cycling, not maintained weight loss. Weight fluctuation is strongly associated with increased risk for diabetes, hypertension, and cardiovascular disease, independent of body weight. In other words, the recommendation to diet may be causing the very diseases it is purported to prevent!"

"There is no magic solution to losing weight and keeping it off in a healthy manner. If you continue to seek the Holy Grail of weight loss, you may be feeling depressed right now. There are no guaranteed solutions — and the commonly recommended methods just aren't showing results."

"The wave of hysteria surrounding obesity can be traced back to many watershed events. In 1986, an NIH consensus panel on obesity ignored nearly all of the data presented to it and declared obesity a serious health threat. It did so despite presentations showing that people who gained weight as they aged reduced their risk of premature death, and that obesity was not related to hardening of the arteries."

"Long-term human studies show that almost all of the excess risk associated with obesity can be accounted for by the higher incidence of weight cycling in obese people, and that obese people with stable weights have very little excess risk."

"Contrary to almost everything you have heard, weight is not a good predictor of health. In fact a moderately active larger person is likely to be far healthier than someone who is svelte but sedentary. Moreover, the efforts of Americans to make themselves thin through dieting and drugs are a major cause of both 'overweight' and the ill health that is wrongly ascribed to it. In other words, America's war on fat is actually helping cause every disease it is supposed to cure."

"There is no good evidence that significant long-term weight loss is beneficial to health, and a great deal of evidence that short-term weight loss followed by weight regain (the pattern followed by almost all dieters) is medically harmful. Indeed, frequent dieting is perhaps the single best predictor of future weight gain."

"Treating cosmetic weight loss as if it were a medical and moral issue tends to make people both considerably fatter and a good deal unhappier than they would otherwise be."

"There is a great deal of evidence that weight LOSS increases the risk for cardiovascular disease among 'overweight' individuals, and some studies suggest that obesity actually protects against vascular disease."

"Glenn Gaesser notes that numerous studies – more than two dozen in the last twenty years alone – have found that weight loss of this magnitude [25 pounds] (and indeed even as little as 10 pounds) leads to an increased risk of premature death, sometimes by an order of several hundred percent. By contrast, during this same time frame only around four studies have found that weight loss leads to lower mortality rates – and one of these found an eleven-hour increase in life expectancy per pound lost."

"The only other large study to look into the question of the health effects of intentional weight loss – the Iowa Women's Health Study – produced some rather extraordinary data in regard to the assumption that trying to get thin is the appropriate 'cure' for the 'disease' of above-average weight. The Iowa study is particularly striking, in that it featured no less than 108 different statistical comparisons, based on age, initial weight and health status, and cause of death. In seventy-nine of these comparisons, intentional weight loss was associated with higher mortality rates. By contrast, the number of comparisons in which intentional weight loss ended up being associated with lower mortality rates was zero. This is especially significant information, given that the Iowa study is one of only a few studies that have distinguished between intentional and unintentional weight loss when measuring the effects of weight loss on health."

"Certain aspects of the medical literature are suggestive, in particular studies that indicate weight cycling (a.k.a. yo-yo dieting) is a major factor in the development of clogged arteries, congestive heart failure, hypertension, and other serious health problems. Indeed, dieters as a group run up to double the risk of developing cardiovascular disease and Type 2 diabetes when compared to 'overweight' people who do not diet. This may be a result of the fact that dieting often leads to bingeing, which is extremely unhealthy, since it is driven by cravings for high-fat, high-sugar foods (indeed, the more often a person diets, the stronger these cravings become). These foods, when consumed by people who have been depriving themselves of adequate caloric intake, are quickly metabolized into visceral body fat, which is far more dangerous to health than subcutaneous fat. (Large people who do not diet tend to have high percentages of subcutaneous fat, but low *percentages of visceral fat. Also, physical activity burns visceral fat very quickly, which helps explain why, as we shall see, activity levels are far more important to health than weight.)"*

"Most groups of people categorized as 'overweight' and 'obese' do not suffer from poorer health or higher mortality than 'ideal weight' individuals. In many of the largest-scale studies, groups of people currently categorized as overweight have better mortality statistics than anyone else. The bulk of the epidemiological evidence suggests that it is more dangerous to be 5 pounds 'underweight' than 75 pounds 'overweight.'"

"From the obesity researchers such as Glenn Gaesser, Paul Ernsberger, Ancel Keys, Reubin Andres, Hilda Bruch, Wayne Callaway, Steven Blair, Elizabeth Barrett-Conner, Janet Polivy, Paul Askew, and Susan Wooley, to eating disorder specialists such as David Garner and Joanne Ikeda, to historians of America's weight obsessions such as Hillel Schwartz and Roberta Seid, to social critics of that obsession such as Richard Klein and Laura Fraser, to feminist critics of our absurdly restrictive body ideal such as Naomi Wolf, Kim Chernin, Susan Bordo, and Susie Orbach, there has been no shortage of erudite and eloquent voices crying out that the case against fat is based on an insidious combination of junk science and cultural neuroses."

"For example, when I asked him to comment on Walter Willett's and Meir Stampfer's recent claim that 'a strong international consensus among scientists' exists that a BMI of 25 and over is a major health risk, obesity researcher Paul Ernsberger pointed out that such claims are based on reports issued by groups like the World Health Organization and the NIH Obesity Task Force. 'The WHO panel consisted entirely of physicians who run weight loss clinics,' he told me. 'Many of these clinics are largely dedicated to prescribing weight loss pills. The NIH Obesity Task Force, as I pointed out in a letter published in JAMA, consisted almost entirely of people running weight loss clinics."

~Paul Campos; *The Obesity Myth*

"It's interesting that clinical trials of weight loss have never shown a longevity benefit, but several clinical trials of weight GAIN show it to be correlated with improved longevity!"
~Paul Ernsberger

To begin with, everything we know about weight loss suggests that losing weight is extremely unhealthy, even if the weight loss is maintained – which it almost never is, and especially when the weight loss is not maintained and the pattern of losing and gaining weight is repeated again and again. But I, and you, should at least be willing to give Paleo the benefit of the doubt. After all, it involves the consumption of a very nutritious, whole foods diet and getting some good exercise in with plenty of time to rest and recover. Even the anti-weight loss authors that I selected recognize that eating a nutritious diet and staying physically fit are generally great virtues (excuse me, I just threw up in my mouth a little as making health recommendations on a statistical basis is kind of my pet peeve).

These lifestyle changes, Paleo-influenced or otherwise, can indeed result in incidental and spontaneous weight loss without a conscious attempt to restrict calories or even macronutrients. As was pointed out in some of the above quotes, there's a difference between unintentional and intentional weight loss. The former is a frequent by-product of an improvement in the healthiness of one's diet, lifestyle, and mindset. The latter comes typically from deliberately limiting one's food intake or burning extra calories through exercise without replacing them with an increase in food intake. And we know that such a strategy does not work out long-term any more than holding your breath to reduce your oxygen levels works out long-term.

"Those who doubt the power of basic drives, however, might note that although one can hold one's breath, this conscious act is soon overcome by the compulsion to breathe. The feeling of hunger is intense and, if not as

potent as the drive to breathe, is probably no less powerful than the drive to drink when one is thirsty. This is the feeling the obese must resist after they have lost a significant amount of weight. The power of this drive is illustrated by the fact that, whatever one's motivation, dieting is generally ineffective in achieving significant weight loss over the long term. The greater the weight loss, the greater the hunger, and, sooner or later for most dieters, a primal hunger trumps the conscious desire to be thin."
~Gina Kolata; *Rethinking Thin*

So I guess what I'm getting at is that weight loss is not just weight loss. And just because a Paleo diet, especially a carbohydrate-restricted Paleo diet, results in spontaneous weight loss – that does not make it healthy. I'm sure that some people who lost weight on the diet did so because the diet and lifestyle was much healthier than what they were pursuing prior. But some didn't. This I know for sure. I've come across many that had to learn the hard way that Paleo, their darling Paleo that they fell in love with when things were going so great – the energy flowed, body fat was flying off, mood was spectacular, was actually causing the new health problems they were encountering (many of them related to hypothyroidism and/or adrenal fatigue).

But you will generally see hypothyroid symptoms emerge with the vast majority of weight loss no matter how that weight loss was achieved – regardless of how unintentional and regardless of how healthy the diet and lifestyle may be. This is due to the simple fact that as body fat stores decline, so does the amount of circulating leptin. As leptin falls, so does thyroid hormone production. Plain and simple, unless of course one happens to increase their sensitivity to leptin hormone – a riddle that modern science has been unable to solve thus far.

But Paleo or not, based on what we know about obesity, one should assume that any weight lost by any means is...

1) Impermanent

2) Unhealthy
3) Destined to trigger health problems attributable to a reduced metabolic rate

Sure, a Paleo diet, when it works for weight loss, is probably one of the highest percentage ways to lose weight without negative repercussion. But that percentage, if I had to estimate, is still probably below 10%.

Most of you will disagree about weight loss being unhealthy. That's because you are confusing assumption for knowledge. There is a big difference. Trust me. I used to "know" it all too. Don't take my word for it. Look into it for yourself. You'll find that once you get past the propaganda promoted by those selling diet books, products, pills, and pet theories that what I have said in this chapter is perhaps more accurate than anything you've ever read on the topic of weight loss

A Quick Primer on How to Overcome Paleo-itis

Well that's that. Other than a lengthy collection of Paleo Horror Stories that I've put together from my site and email inbox, that's the gist of my Paleo criticism. I hope it was enough to open your mind to other possibilities. That's all I ask and all I was attempting to do. If you think this connection between nutrition and human health is a closed case, or that we know everything there is to know about how to use nutrition to conquer disease, please keep it to yourself. All of these naïve panacea pissing contests are getting in the way of people living their lives, and instill in people a sense of false hope again and again – each failure more soul-crushing than the last.

But I will wrap this up with a few simple pointers on how to get your health and metabolism back on track if you did experience some problems on a Paleo diet (or any diet really). The first is to take your morning body temperature. It should be at least 98 degrees F when you first wake up in the morning. If it is not, this is a prime indicator that your body is conserving energy. This may be a new development or a lifelong condition. Odds are, following the Paleo diet probably didn't do your metabolism any favors – particularly if you were restricting carbohydrates on top of it. Now, if you are a hard-training athlete, low body temperature comes with the territory. But for a normal person with no reason to be conserving energy, this is an important warning sign of dysfunction taking place on the inside. You don't want your body conserving energy. You want everything firing on all cylinders and living life at max capacity.

This too, is no panacea. More of a quick jumpstart to get yourself back on track. But it almost always at least helps to improve mood, digestion, the warmth of hands and feet, menstrual irregularities, hypoglycemia, irritability, anxiety, insomnia, low sex drive, poor hair and nail growth, and dozens of other things that can be adversely impacted by a suboptimal metabolism. I won't list them all here. *Hypothyroidism Type 2* author Mark Starr's chapter on the symptoms of a low metabolism is 85 pages long if that's any indication!

While I'm not an advocate of "junk food," per se, and I do recognize the importance of a nutritious diet comprised of mostly unadulterated, unprocessed foods long-term, there is no question that the most useful weapon against a low metabolism is the calorie. Unprocessed foods make it difficult to truly get in enough calories. If you think you can without having to resort to processed foods, more power to you. But many simply can't, or lack the digestive prowess to even extract enough material from the unprocessed food that they are eating.

To prove my point, I ate a 3-pound bag of potatoes yesterday. That's about 25 golf-ball sized potatoes. And well, that's still not even quite 1,000 calories. To someone who has been starving themselves for years, well sure. That may sound like a lot of calories. But during recovery I like to see most males getting 4,000-5,000 calories per day and most women

3,000-4,000 – until body temperature has reached 98 degrees F. Consume less than that and you prolong the amount of time that you will suffer from health problems related to a low metabolism – if you ever get there at all. That's just reality. So now what are you going to do? Eat 15 pounds of potatoes to get all your calories? Good luck.

For that reason, I like to see people doing a complete 180 (heh heh) on their strict healthy diet that caused so many health problems, and quickly fix their health problems eating pizza, cheeseburgers, pie, ice cream, and pretty much whatever else sounds delicious. It's usually what sounds the best that instigates the largest calorie consumption. And what sounds the best is usually what your body needs the most to shut down stress hormones and increase metabolism giant leaps at a time. Variety is huge too, from meal to meal and from day to day. A typical buffet is the ultimate pro-metabolism playground.

This is not a permanent thing. The more you just go for it, the more quickly you recover. Then you can return to eating a more normal, maintenance amount of calories and consume more unprocessed foods. To give you an example of how quickly it can happen, a woman who I've been working with one-on-one recently went from roughly 96 degrees F to 99 degrees F in just 3 weeks, and no that's not a fever she's running.

Other helpful tips:

- Do not restrict any macronutrient, but emphasize carbohydrates, followed by fat (saturated being the best – from red meat, dairy products, and coconut), followed by protein – especially if you have been doing the opposite for months or years. Remember that you will be getting lots of protein from foods other than meat and your protein requirements will be lessened in a caloric surplus

- Eat tons of salt and don't drink too many fluids – keeping some good color to your urine and not letting it get clear or pale yellow is a tremendous help when restoring metabolism, especially for those who truly have a low metabolism, which usually triggers frequent urination and very clear urine
- If you feel your hands and feet get cold or feel a sudden urge to urinate, or urinate several times in a short duration with clear urine, eat a nice salty snack like cheese and saltine crackers, potato chips, salted peanuts, pretzels, salty popcorn, or something else that you might be served while sitting on a plane
- Don't exercise at all
- Sleep as much as you possibly can
- Eat as much food as you can within 30 minutes of waking up each day, and eat heavier at breakfast and lunch than you do at dinner

In other words, obey the five S's of metabolism…
- Sleep
- Starch
- Sugar
- Salt
- Saturated fat

And utter this phrase to yourself or out loud, preferably out loud, whenever you sit down to eat something that you think might be bad for you or that you are afraid to eat…
"I eat like a Badass!"
Or the alternate…"I eat like a Boss!" (Boss should be pronounced to rhyme with house or mouse).

If you want MUCH more thorough (albeit general) information about the importance of metabolism, how it shuts down, how to restore it, and how to heal your relationship with food, read my book *Diet Recovery 2*.

I'm Matt Stone. I hope you enjoyed reading this book. Remember boys and girls…

EAT THE FOOD!

Paleo Fails

Here is an overwhelmingly large collection of stories that people have sent to me documenting their failures on a Paleo-inspired diet and lifestyle. These people are not professional writers, although some probably should be! Some of their experiences are valid and some are not – where they are thinking that their problems were caused by Paleo but perhaps were not. These stories are not all necessarily meant to be valid criticism of the Paleo diet. But, for whatever reason, these people felt the need to share these stories in hopes of rescuing someone just like them, experiencing similar problems, and unable to get unstuck with their beliefs that the Paleo diet, if they could just endure long enough, would deliver them the health they sought after.

I have not edited these stories at all other than correcting flagrant grammatical and spelling errors. I occasionally add a little commentary in **Bold** for clarification when needed.

If you are struggling on Paleo, you might find some of these stories sounding eerily familiar to your own. Enjoy…

Paleo Messes with Your Body and Your Head

By: Corey Friese

It was July of 2008 when I decided to give up the SAD I had been consuming and start being more conscious of my health. I started reading Dr. Mercola's website and concluded I was a "protein type" and that my recommended foods were beef, eggs, other meats, and non-starchy vegetables. Sounds familiar eh? It kind of sounds like any other "paleo" or "primal" diet that is labeled as the natural diet of man.

When I started eating a high fat/protein diet, I felt amazing. It seemed all my health ails were vanishing. Acne, cloudy mind, lack of energy, vitality was soaring it seemed. Different variations of this way of eating came and went (Zero Carb, Meat and vegetables, etc.). All of it was very low in carbohydrate, maybe <30g a day. The zero carb obviously being pure meat and eggs. Lots of muscle meat too. Carbohydrates were taboo for me, absolutely no sugar/starch. I remember eating a small sweet potato one night after being carb-restricted for a while and had my blood sugar spike to an insane level. I can see how the low-carb crowd chastises them as their bodies are in such a different state that they cannot handle them when consumed even in small quantities, ala your Snickers bar and subsequent forehead eruption. **(This is a personal anecdote I had shared years ago – eating a high-fat diet for a long period of time caused me to have severe acne breakouts eating things that used to not give me problems at all prior).**

I kept to this path for quite some time and like others, was under the impression that I had uncovered the secret or panacea to optimal health. Boy was I wrong! I gradually lost my sex drive, was tremendously underweight, and had skin issues come back. I was a mental wreck too. My cortisol levels were definitely through the roof. I was making irrational decisions in my life, was stressed, and always felt awkward with friends because I was never able to just chill out and drink a beer!

My road to recovery first began with adding starch to my diet. That helped a lot. I eventually stagnated and only until I introduced tremendous amounts of simple sugars did everything really start coming back. Sex drive, ability to exercise and lift weights, skin is clear, and especially: my sanity is back! I now have anywhere from 500-800g of carbohydrates every day. I drink soda, I eat hamburgers from Burger King, basically anything and everything (especially gluten-laden products, which used to be a big problem for me) and feel great now. I can vouch and testify to the fact that a low-carb/paleo diet definitely messes with not only your body but your head too. Instructions for meat exclusive eaters: Go out and buy a pizza and a bottle of soda, it will free you.

Have You Been Seduced by the Paleo Narrative?

By Thomas Seay

The Paleo diet has a seductive narrative that makes it appealing, even irresistible. It goes like this: our distant ancestors ate a certain way. Genetically we haven't changed much since then. Therefore we should eat as they did. You throw in the *Encyclicals* from a few of the High Bishops of Paleo- "The Gary", Dr. Harris, Chris Kresser, Loren Cordain, Emily Dean, etc.- lending scientific gravitas- and you have yourself a **myth**. Perhaps you don't recognize them as Encyclicals because they are written on "blogs" instead of parchment. By myth, I do not mean "false", "fabrication". By myth, I mean a story you live by. A story or principles around which you organize meaning, a lens through which you see the world. I like the story physicist Michio Kaku tells about how as a child he used to imagine fish scientists (in the pond at that San Francisco Golden Gate Park Japanese Tea Garden) who were creating theories of the world based upon everything being submerged in water. Everybody has a myth. Everybody. Even the most "scientific" person. ESPECIALLY the most scientific person!

A lot of people are living the Paleo myth and that's fine, if it's working for you: namely, you are truly maintaining good health. The problem with myths is that they can fail you and you are so submerged in them (like the fish scientists) that you can't see beyond them. There is at least a comfort that comes from the certainty they provide.

Now I've got to tell you. I have been seduced by the Paleo narrative, but it's time to throw it off. *I have fared dismally on the Paleo diet.* Mind you, when I began this experiment I was not overweight. I have eaten healthy for a long, long time, so I did not come to this screwed up from a SAD diet. *However, the negative results from this diet (for me, I must qualify) have been dramatic.* Despite having come to this conclusion about two weeks ago, when I think about it, sometimes a voice whispers to me, "...what would your Paleolithic ancestors have done?"

And here is Thomas in a comment vs. something he wrote on a public site as a post (www.paleohacks.com). As you can see it's a little more loose, direct, to the point, and friggin' hilarious (FH)…

Paleo sucks. Here are a few vignettes from my 8 month Paleo ODyssey.

Ever take your kite out to the park, only to find there was no wind? Then you try running as hard as you can, but the damn thing still won't fly? That was My Penis on Paleo. It should be called the "Anti-Boner Diet". If you have plans on becoming a celibate monk, it just might be the diet for you. Good news: problem resolved immediately upon adding plenty of carbs back in.

Wait a minute. Not only will it help you if you don't want to have sex, it will also help you if you don't ever want to shit again. Here's a true story. One day I was sitting on the pot, thinking I could crap (after I don't know how many days). However, the shit would not come out of my ass. I sat there for 40 minutes. It felt like my rectum was going to explode because there was so much shit accumulated that would not come out. I SERIOUSLY considered calling 9-1-1. I thought I was going to rupture something. There was blood. Finally I drank some hot water and magnesium and got it out. Now I have had constipation before, but nothing like this.

And then there was the stress. Now I sometimes have a stressful job as a Software Engineer, but actually the period during which I was doing Paleo was rather quiet in terms of my career. Nonetheless I was constantly on edge while doing this diet. Again, immediately resolved once I switched to higher carbs.

Lauren

I started eating Low-Carb Paleo in August of 2010 after trying veganism out for a month and a half. As a low-fat, low-sugar vegan, I was practically a walking zombie. I ate mostly whole grains and vegetables. I lost about 5 pounds during my vegan stage and also stopped getting my period. I was happy to lose the weight because I had gained ten pounds by eating lots of naturally-sweetened desserts between 2009 and 2010. This is not to say I was anywhere near overweight: when I decided to go vegan I weighed about 127 pounds and was 5'7. I have had strong perfectionist tendencies throughout my life and I didn't like the changes my body went through as I grew up. I wanted to be 110 pounds and modelesque.

In August 2010, my mom's doctor suggested the Paleo diet for her chronic fatigue. She ordered a popular book about the diet and I read it in one day. I believed what the book said about nutrition and the fattening properties of all carbohydrates. I switched to a meat-, nut-, fruit-, and vegetable-heavy diet. I dropped down to 117 pounds and stayed around 115-120 from August 2010 to June 2011, my year of Paleo eating. During that time, also my sophomore year of college, I experienced an array of health and psychological issues. I became quite fearful and neurotic about eating only "good" food (organic, pastured, paleo-approved, whatever).

By my first week of school I started getting head colds and viruses nearly every two weeks. I didn't have time for anything besides schoolwork and cooking meals from scratch (endless hours of vegetable washing were involved). I wouldn't eat out practically anywhere except for an organic restaurant downtown, and when I ate there I would feel guilty for eating mashed sweet potato. The horror! I was anxious and sick all the time. I regularly saw a holistic doctor who encouraged my controlling eating habits which I now believe were an eating disorder. My hair started falling out in January 2011. I continued eating Low Carb and experimented with Zero Carb (extremely high fat- sometimes 200g/day) as well as Intermittent Fasting. At this point, around April/May 2011 I was down to 115 pounds and actually happy about it. My body and face looked much less feminine than a year prior (in my opinion), but I was happy to have what I considered and acceptable number on the scale. I also started getting tonsil stones around this time- Google them if you wish. They're gross.

In May of 2011 I visited a gynecologist to see what she thought of my Amenorrhea (lack of a menstrual period). I had been seeing the holistic doctor since November 2010 for this reason but had not seen any positive progress in my hormonal health throughout the year. She said that my lack of period was likely from stress or low body fat. She said I was underweight at 115 pounds and 5'7.25". Blood tests and ultrasounds showed that my thyroid was normal, Progesterone was a bit low, and Estrogen was quite low. I was told to eat more fat (not what I needed- I was eating 180g/day) to gain weight. I took gaining weight seriously, though, and incorporated nice doses of carbohydrates in the form of butternut squash and sweet potato into my diet. Within 6 weeks I gained 8 pounds and grew 0.75". I also started seeing an acupuncturist regularly who helped me work out a lot of psychological stuff and gain confidence.

I worked hard to gain my health and sanity back over the summer. In September 2011 I finally started my period again. I bravely began eating at restaurants and trying foods that the holistic doctor convinced me I was allergic to through muscle testing. These foods include wheat and sugar. So far I have only seen good things come from not being afraid of ANY types of foods. I allow myself to eat pretty much anything in reasonable amounts, including processed foods and desserts. I try to maintain balance in my diet and I love eating out with friends. I am free to socialize and travel more now that my diet is flexible. My digestion has been getting stronger and the constipation/constant gnawing cramp in my intestines has disappeared. I am MUCH calmer and happier.

At 5'8" I weigh about 135 pounds and to be honest I am not completely content with my body image yet (I can't remember a time in my life when I have been, regardless of my weight). That is what I still have to work on: accepting my looks and not letting them cause me distress. It's embarrassing and shallow, but I still get upset about having gained weight sometimes. I am starting to see myself more realistically, though. I recognize that I have gained weight in attractive places (hips, bust, not much in the waist) and look much more womanly now. I am slowly getting more comfortable with this new body. I just need to let go of trying to look like a Victoria's Secret model because it is clear that my health is much better at this weight than it would be at 110 pounds.

Just as I am still getting healthier psychologically, I continue to make gains in my physical health. My immune system is not yet back to where it was before my Paleo year. I still get sick more often than I would like to- maybe once every two months. But I've noticed that getting sick doesn't debilitate me very much because I am physically stronger and less obsessed with being healthy. Getting sick used to mean I was "failing" in some way. I've let go of that silly notion. I expect that my immune system will continue to improve, just as my psychological and hormonal health continue to.

I urge anyone who reads about Paleo or any other diet to be cautious. If something drastic happens when you try a diet, like loss of period or hair, you should probably stop or change what you're doing. If you are trying to reach some image of perfection, remember that true health isn't perfection. True health is made up of balance, sanity, lack of sickness, and happiness. Be gentle with yourself. Don't go to extremes, even though our friend Matt Stone has learned a lot from doing so ☺. And if you do go to extremes, expect consequences.

Andrew

I followed the Mark Sisson primal/paleo regime for about 2 years. In the beginning I lost 25 pounds and felt great. I thought I'd found the "right" way to live. It took about 8 months for things to start going wrong. I started getting head colds. My energy and mood sucked. At first I just wrote it off as the typical winter cold. Unfortunately it blossomed into a full blown sinus infection that I struggled with off and on for an entire semester. Things deteriorated from there. I became cranky, irritable, and prone to fits of anger. For the first time in my life I began experiencing panic attacks. Everyday stresses became overwhelming. My sleep suffered tremendously. This was perhaps the most damaging part of low-carb paleo for me. I wouldn't sleep for days at a time, and if I did sleep it was only for an hour or two. The insomnia and stress took its toll on my health. I went from 170 lbs to 195. My hair began thinning rapidly and my skin blemished.

Finally, my brother convinced me to look into a few blogs, including Matt's 180 Degree Health and Stephen Guyenet's Whole Health Source. I read Matt's ebook on Diet Recovery and was relieved to find that my experience with paleo wasn't uncommon. I stopped fearing carbs and started eating potatoes, bread, and rice and took a break from exercise. I've noticed gradual improvements ever since. My skin is clearer, my sleep is more regular, and I'm back to being an easy-going guy again. My fiancé calls me a space-heater because I'm putting off so much heat at times. It's not perfect though, I still struggle with insomnia and stress. Most nights I need two slices of white bread just to fall asleep. But things look better than they have in a long time. Thanks Matt.

Thor Falk

I have recently tried a period of very low-carb diet, and I had some pretty unpleasant side effects in the form of palpitations bordering on an arrhythmia of the heart, and I finally got around collecting my thoughts on this.

To put this in context – palpitations are not entirely unusual for me. Funnily enough I suspected for a long time that they are at least in part related to not eating (as sometimes I got them whenever I had not eaten for a long time, and as soon as I ate something it became better).

Thanks to my recent experiment I think I now understand it better: I am pretty sure that they are related to not eating enough carbs, and more precisely to a situation where my body is in ketosis (which does make sense, as the heart can only run on carbs or on ketone bodies).

It all started maybe two weeks after I had gone low-carb paleo, with 50-100g carbs per day whilst training pretty heavily, both HIIT and weights. At one point I started having palpitations, and they were particularly heavy during periods of max heartrate (and/or when the heartrate came down too quickly in fact). So if ever you wondered why I stopped the testosterone "density" workouts (or any of the other hormone specific workouts for that matter) – the reason was simply that they did not feel right with palpitations becoming too strong, especially on high frequency overhead-pressing exercises for some strange reason.

I had read somewhere that palpitations could be related to a VLC diet (I did start a thread on Mark Sisson's forum at the time) and I learned that a VLC diet could lead to a potassium / magnesium imbalance, so I decided to (a) eat loads of bananas, and (b) supplement K & Mg. Unfortunately to no avail.

Then along came Kurt Harris' Paleo 2.0 article, and I learned that some Paleo folk are not that negative on starches, as long as they come from rice and/or potatoes. I decided to give it a try – so I at one meal of rice (maybe 25g of carbs), and a meal of potatoes (maybe 50g of carbs) on the next day, in addition to the carbs I would be eating anyway (fruits, vegetables, dairy, 85% chocolate). Funnily enough, the palpitations stopped pretty much immediately and did not return for the last 10 days or so.

So my take-away: VLC is not for everyone – some people might just experience a carb-flu, but for some people (eg myself) things can get a bit more serious. Maybe eventually I would get over it, but I am not sure I want to try again…

John

Funny…most of the Paleo people immediatley assume those that failed on the diet weren't eating correctly. I was eating only "Paleo-approved" things and spent a fortune on only grass-fed meats, raw organic nuts and seeds, cage free eggs, etc., and had a great time of it at first…then ran into most of the issues cited by many users on here. Eating natural carbs again from rice, corn, and potatoes totally saved me…getting my body temperature back up was huge. Glad you are open-minded to reading opposing opinions though! Such opinions are always appreciated!

Sheila

I have seen quite a few folks in my practice and social circle try Paleo – they always get high as a kite, essentially manic, and then crash if they push it too far (as in keep at it longer than they should). I like to remind those who will listen of Dr. Schwarzbein's illustrative metaphor that spending feels great, saving is boring, but we have to do both to be balanced.

Lee

Matt, here is my testimonial. The Paleo Diet made me an internet blog reading slut.

IGD

I lost my bloody hair on paleo and looked sick like a sub saharan skeleton! NO THANKS!

Rob

I was a vegan for five and a half years, for ethical and environmental reasons. I started reading about the paleo diet during that time, and became a philosophical convert, and it took me a while to start eating meat after becoming convinced that humans were not 'natural vegans' as I'd long maintained. It took several years before I could get around to 'doing what I needed,' which was to eat a Nora Gedgaudas style, grain free, ketogenic, high fat, lowish protein diet. It seemed to make sense- fat produces an even energy stream, a log on the fire instead of the paper or kindling that carbs represented. That's why you don't need to eat as often or as much- your fat burning adaptation allowed you not to be a slave to putting wood on the fireplace.

I did eat sweet potatoes, the beloved starch of paleo advocates, but usually not more than one a day. And I did feel good- better, more even energy, probably a small bit of fat loss, and freedom from the swings of hypoglycemia.

But within a couple of months, I ran into some trouble. For one, I would wake up in the middle of the night, heart racing, unable to sleep. I would finally fall back asleep after a few hours, just in time to feel groggy and awful when my day started. Also, I would oddly get crazy blood sugar drops when I ate a shake at night. I couldn't figure out why a coconut milk, raw milk, egg yolk, handful of frozen berry meal would throw me for a loop. (Reactive hypogycemia, perhaps?). **(This is very common with liquid meals – even drinking too many fluids will cause this, or eating lots of fruit – I don't think it's hypoglycemia in the strict sense, but a mild version of water intoxication/hyponatremia).**

But the biggest and most debilitating part was the toll it took on me socially. I could barely go to events without concern about whether the 'right' kind of food would be there. If I went to a potluck, I'd eat around the edges of salads or maybe some meat, but mostly just feel frustrated and unhappy. I had become even more crazy than I was before about diet, and just couldn't figure out why so many people in the world had gotten it so, so wrong. The final straw was the toll it took on garden planning in the house I was a part of- don't grow corn, or potatoes, but sweet taters were sort of ok, and squash too maybe. Mainly, I wanted cabbage and broccoli and cauliflower and above ground leafy vegetables. If you're a gardener, you know those generally suck as calorie sources compared to roots and grains.

Anyway, I found Matt and 180 Health. We corresponded, and he had helpful words for me. Here was a guy who'd read all the books I had, and all the books I wanted to read, and somehow was advocating something besides what I thought they had resoundingly established. Better pay attention, I thought. He suggested trusting our appetite and cravings, not seeing the body as trying to sabotage our well-being. He was in favor of a sensible, whole foods based diet, but also put on a premium on de-stressing and climbing out of the trap of orthorexia.

I started loosening up my diet, not freaking out so much. It's a couple years later, and I'm getting the hang of it. I really resonate with the observation that just about everyone I've encountered who's really into some stripe of 'healthy eating' has mediocre health, at best. And with the stress and social isolation I experienced when it was me against the crazy non-vegan, non-paleo world, I can see why.

To paleo eaters, or potential paleo eaters: the idea has some merit and resonance. I still recognize that grain agriculture has been a driving force in desertification and ecological destruction throughout its history. The emphasis on grass-based, regenerative animal agriculture among many paleos is admirable and important. Given its small share of the market, I think it's worth supporting those farmers regularly. And while I'm skeptical that we know the full story when it comes to antinutrients in seed foods (phytic acid may supposedly have anticancer effects, and I wouldn't be surprised if other 'antinutrients' had as yet unforeseen benefits alongside their detriments), there's probably no harm in experimenting with other carbs beside wheat and corn and rice, which provide the lion's share of the world's calories. Simply from a balance perspective, branching out makes sense to me. The paleo framework is also a good one to filter other ideas through, like those related to movement, or education, or child-raising. But it's hard to say with certainty how we ate or lived way back in the time before writing, and I think it's also a fallacy to think that it's all been a mis-step somehow, and we need only to get back to the right, timeless path.

Rather than look back at the failures behind us and think we're at the end of history, I like to look ahead and imagine we're just getting started with history. Agriculture and animal husbandry had far-reaching consequences that we're just now starting to understand, and navigating what lies before us is the start of a new story. In that frame, a hard line paleo ideology is just putting our heads into the sand. Better to grapple with the questions and contradictions than retreat from them, in my mind.

And with that, good luck and happy eating!

B.K.

I can't believe that in all my years of researching and wondering that I never figured out that all that feeling was was my adrenal glands, doing their darndest to keep me afloat during the apparent food shortage I was living through. Duh! Of course! And a "runners high?" What the hell is that? I know so many runners who babble on and on about it as if it's the sign that what they're doing is good for them, never mind the shin splits and torn tendons…And I would feel the same whenever I'd do a fun little fast. See! I feel good! Proof positive that what I'm doing is a source of a totally natural high, and boy oh boy, if it's a "natural" reaction of the body, it MUST be healthy! Ha! How stupid! As if it's all just simple input-output! I bet Jesus felt pretty fucking spiritual after forty days in the desert without food. I bet when the devil came by to tempt him into some bread making magic, Jesus was so far into his all-natural catecholamine high that he just laughed him off.

So anyway, I starved myself on and off throughout my teenage years, but then as my twenties dawned I took on a more respectable approach and would periodically cut out carbs. But then, disaster struck: After many years of physical and emotional stress (my family is so screwed up that they truly take the fun OUT of dysfunction. Dysction, I guess.) I got weirdly ill. My knee was so messed up that until the MRI showed no actual tissue damage, the doctor thought I had ruptured my ACL. A similar mystery happened to my foot, I started losing weight without trying, had huge dark circles under my eyes, spasms and twitches all over my body, my heart rate and blood pressure would shoot sky high at random, my hair was coming out in clumps and what was growing in was super baby fine, my hands and feet and shins tingled all the time, I had gross yellow-green bruises everywhere, burns and cuts took forever to heal…and I am eating a really healthy diet at this point.

So I go to a million doctors and they think there's nothing wrong, I need a vacation or something. Hot dog! I really felt like traveling! I couldn't get out of bed! And I was uninsured, blowing through all my savings to pay my medical bills AND I had to give up my job! Yeah! I'll take a fucking cruise! Thanks Doc! After awhile they started prescribing Valium. I just could not believe that the random spikes in my heart rate were anxiety attacks. I would be fine, reading a book, laughing at a joke, and then BAM. Heart rate spike. Start sweating, getting really cold…I was waking up drenched in cold sweats, I mean, this was awful! So I searched and searched for an answer and then I encountered the Lyme community. Anyone familiar with these guys? Pretty much the idea is that if you have a weird problem that's gone undiagnosed, you have Lyme, as well as a few other tick-born pathogens, most likely.

I don't mean to say that this theory isn't possibly the truth for many, but the way these "Lyme Literate M.D's" approach it is a joke. I went to this doctor and he asked me if I had been experiencing "fatigue and malaise." Why yes doctor! Indeed I have! "Okay!" he says "You have Lyme!" and he proceeds to write me THREE scripts for THREE different antibiotics, all of which I'm supposed to take for six months, all at the same time. And when I asked him questions, when I asked to have the diagnosis explained, my skepticism was sort of swatted away with a puzzled look and, wait for it, a prayer. He prayed for my healing....but I'm going online and all these really desperate people are so glad to get help, and a lot of these Lyme stories sound like me...but I'm way too freaked by the inevitable fallout of such a protocol that I hold off on the antibiotics and go on an all-natural approach instead.

So I decided on a low carb modified paleo that allowed a bit of dairy. Maybe not paleo so much as early shepherding nomad man, mainly because germs love sugar so I figured I'd starve them to death. That's always an interesting theory, that germs need sugar to live so stop eating sugar...I know of another organism that needs sugar to live too...hmmm. Anyway, the only fruit I ate was green apples because I figured they were probably the closest commercially available thing to the sour, knotted fruits that grow wild here in the temperate zone...I ate sweet potatoes occasionally...I just ate tons and tons of meat. Craving a cracker?? I'll just fry up some chicken thighs real crispy to give it that crackery crunch! Mmm mmm! Still hungry?!!? Even after eating all that delicious, nourishing protein??? How 'bout three avocados and a head of raw cabbage! What's this? Digestive upset?? HOW? Think of all the ENZYMES from those delicious raw vegetables!!! Think about how HEALTHY it is to eat vegetables that aren't really that tasty, have no quantifiable caloric value and are trying their darndest to keep animals like us from eating them! Yum! What's this? You say I can have UNLIMITED RAW VEGGIES???? Oh happy day! Really, I just love to eat veggies. They're my favorite food, I swear, no I never crave processed foods like cake! HA HA! Ha. ha.

Anyway, I did this for about four months, along with swallowing down a ton of "immune boosting" or rather, "putting your immune system into hyper-overdrive" supplements. I was losing more and more weight (to note, one doctor told me I looked "good" since the precipitous, unintended weight loss), literally literally literally my skin thinned out. I could see all my blood vessels in gross detail, WATER hurt my hands. Bathing was a real challenge. The only thing that made me feel normal for about twenty minutes was coffee. I know, real Paleo. Well who knows, when did the South American Indians start drinking coffee? Is coffee allowed on Paleo? I just know it has no sugar, so I was good to go. And I'd feel like myself for a brief window in time, and then it was back to bed.

During this low carb bout, my blood pressure sunk from a lifetime average of 135/80 to 95/70....When a nurse took my BP and saw this, I gasped and explained to her that never in my life had my BP been that low...she just looked at me like I was crazy and assured me that low blood pressure is a good thing! Well, what about the fact that I'm thinner now than I was as an enthusiastic intravenous drug user, even though I'm housing bunless burgers at every opportunity?? "Great!" she smiles, "Weight loss is great, you're within a normal range for your height, you look great!" Well, what about the fact that I almost passed out three times since I've been sitting here with you, nurse? "GREAT! Most Americans BP and weight is high, so if yours is drastically lower, then that has to be a good thing! Cuz high is bad and low is good! Of course! Now sit tight, the doctor will be right in to further ignore these alarming numbers!" (She didn't say the last line.)

So, long story short(ened an bit), after a while I gave up the whole theory and found a cheap doctor right down the road from my house who cursed and fist bumped and was actually open to there being something wrong with me other than needing to go to Disneyland or having an unprovable tick disease…and I also lied to him and told him that Addison's disease runs in my family just to get him to test my adrenals because I had read that doctors never do so on their own. Sure enough, my catecholamines were undetectably low, as tested via a 24 hour whizz test and blood work. No epiniephrine, no dopamine, and scant amounts of cortisol. I was checked out for tumors and growths and other weird stuff that could cause this, and I checked out clear for all of them. To my doctor, it's still a mystery, but to me, I knew exactly what the problem was. I had seriously blown the shit out of my adrenals, and I did it through stress, and very large part of that stress being dietary, dietary like eating a pile of meat and vegetables and treating myself to a sour apple for dessert. Mmm.

I retooled my whole approach, ate an organic scoop of vanilla ice cream on a sugar cone with rainbow sprinkles daily, stopped most of the supplements, but I started taking minerals and amino acids (to help with the dopamine) a B complex for adrenal support as well as maca, holy basil, and licorice to help with cortisol production, E to help with circulation. I stopped the coffee, stopped feeling bad about needing to lay in bed and made sure to never ever ever let myself get hungry. Food on me at all times. Within a month the circles were fading from under my eyes, the spasms and twitches were almost history, water no longer stung to the touch and I was able to go for a mile long walk without having to turn around. What a triumph it was. I'm still not 100 % (this was a fairly recent ordeal),but I am much improved. I truly thought I was going to die if I didn't figure out what the hell the problem was, and I'm very glad I did. Perhaps if I had been reading the 180 blog instead of the Lyme people or the Paleo people's blogs, I'd have felt better a lot sooner.

I really like what you're doing here, I think you're documenting a journey of thought and that you're coming to the realization that most of the secrets of health are hidden in plain sight. And to all those who are all mad at you and want diet plans and statistics, they are missing the entire point and I don't think it's something you can convince them of. People have to realize it for themselves.

Everything has trade offs. Grains and dairy can make you fat, sure. But they can also make you healthy, fertile, taller and stronger, as our evolution and history proves. Demonizing food groups that took us from squat, compact, short-lived beasts to the overpopulated, comfortable mess we are now is a short-sighted point of view. And if you really need an argument for why civilized foods are okay, perhaps you haven't been subjected to a good cheese board lately, hmmm?

In

My experience is too disjointed to draw many conclusions on how paleo affected me, however, this much I am pretty sure of. The anti-carb propaganda did very much affect my choices. Furthermore, I am much calmer and handle stress a lot better eating more carbs. It's more convenient, I feel better, more socially acceptable – all of which makes low carb/paleo stupid and unworkable for me.

You and your blog is what finally got me thinking differently about the whole low-carb/paleo notion (and about health ideologies in general). That the positive benefits noticed (which is why it is convincing) are not long term, that fat metabolism is potentially stressful, I could go on and on.

I feel like I owe you and wanted to chime in and thank you. You positively influenced me on this point. I think you do great stuff here and have one of the (if not the) most insightful and interesting health blogs.

Luke

Here is my story. I tried to keep it as related to low-carb paleo as I could.

Getting sick is easy. All you have to do is read some books and websites on health and nutrition, create rules for eating based on what you think is "good" or "bad", and follow those rules at all costs even when your body screams at you to stop. One of the most harmful rules I ever adopted was the "carbohydrates are bad, or at least suboptimal from a longevity and health standpoint" rule. This rule was based on the belief that our paleolithic ancestors did not have access to significant amounts of carbohydrates and so they subsisted mostly on fat, protein, and non-starchy and non-sweet carbohydrates.

The first dietary decision guided by this rule was to remove all grains from my diet. Over the course of a few years I went through periods of temporarily avoiding other carb sources like fruit and dairy while eating a predominantly raw food diet that included ample amounts of animal products, fats, vegetables, and all the other "paleo" foods. I acknowledged that most of my foods would not have been found in the wild habitats of my paleolithic ancestors, but my intention was to approximate the macronutrient ratios that I believed were ideal. For the first few years after having gradually shifted from SAD to a mostly raw paleo diet I felt great. Benefits included clearer skin, more energy, better digestion, the ability to easily gain weight, a very light and clear feeling often associated with raw diets, and lessening of asthma symptoms. I was 18 years old at the time I started experimenting with diet, and I didn't have any major health problems to begin with, aside from cat dander-induced asthma (which diet never healed). So my intention was to become even healthier.

I wasn't too strict about avoiding carbs in the beginning, but upon noticing the development of some dental caries after eating lots of fresh summer berries, and having experienced many blood sugar swings from eating too much fruit, I decided to largely eliminate fruit from my diet. I figured I could get all of those nutrients from vegetables and without the sugar. My teeth stopped getting worse. Around that time, I was experimenting with intermittent fasting and alternate day fasting. I loved the focused feeling fasting gave me. It was strikingly similar to the effects of a cup of coffee, like slow-release coffee, which I now realize was due to my adrenals pumping out extra stress hormones in response to the lack of food. Also around that time I started to notice my hair was falling out more than usual and was changing its texture. There were other minor changes like dandruff, brief periods of poor digestion and gas, inability to focus, and low energy.

After I graduated from college I started working a full time job-that I hated, which was a major source of stress. I would bike to and from work and I would often skip lunch. I was eating very few carbs. At that time, I started to experience more digestive problems which included lots of diarrhea and incomplete digestion of foods in general. I found it increasingly difficult to focus especially in the stressful environment of work and couldn't think clearly. My brain wasn't working well, and I felt like I was getting dumber. I was extremely emotional. My energy fluctuated greatly throughout the day, and I was exhausted most of the time. I wasn't sleeping well and having very strange dreams when I did sleep. My health fell apart over the period of a few months. In response to these health problems, I switched from eating mostly raw foods to mostly cooked foods, which seemed to digest better and not make me feel as ill when I ate them. At one point I ran out of money and was living on free potatoes and vegetables from a farmer's market along with some high-quality organ meats and coconut oil. I had been avoiding carbs entirely except for a little fruit and so my body did not handle the starch in the sweet potatoes well. I had more bouts of diarrhea and all my problems worsened.

At that time I realized I had some serious gut dysbiosis, despite drinking copious amounts of EM probiotics and eating the standard list of fermented foods so popular among WAP folk, and so I thought the solution was to go even lower carb. After all, my symptoms got much worse when I tried to eat potatoes or if I ate too much fruit, and all the candida fear mongerers said starches and sugars were the problem. It made sense at the time. So I ate nothing but fat (butter and coconut oil by the spoon), animals (mostly organ meats, bone marrow, stocks/broths, and other WAP-type foods of the low-carb variety), and cooked vegetables. I eliminated all dairy (except for butter) and all sugars and starches. After about three weeks of this diet all my digestive issues completely went away. My energy was way better, my skin was perfectly clear, and my hair stopped falling out. I did notice that I would have heart palpitations every night, and that cuts on my fingers would get infected and take a very long time to heal, and that I was peeing like crazy around noon and throughout the night, but those problems were minor compared to the major digestive disturbances I was experiencing before.

I began to read stories similar to mine, and I knew that carbohydrates were not the root of my problem. Besides, I used to eat all the carbs I wanted before I was concerned with this nutrition stuff and I felt great. Something had changed in my body and it could no longer effectively utilize carb-rich foods. I started to reconceptualize what health meant. Health is what I had when I was a kid — a robust body that can handle a wide variety of foods, a reservoir of energy. Health is not avoiding a bunch of "bad" foods and attaining a magical state of dietary perfection.

So I began eating more carbs, and slowly my health problems returned. They returned with a vengeance. Since eliminating all carbs helped me before, I tried it again out of desperation, but my condition worsened with this second attempt. I couldn't digest anything, I couldn't focus, and often I felt so bad I didn't want to interact with other people. My heart would race and my brain would fog after every meal I ate. My lymphatic system was clogged up to the point of pain. I'm sure I was on my way to ulcerative colitis. With every diet I tried and every rule I followed, low-carb or high-carb or whatever, my health worsened, aside from temporary improvements in some areas. I lost all trust in my mental ideas about health and diet because each one failed me miserably, and certainly, no external authority could tell me how to get healthy.

So what was the alternative? I abandoned everything I thought I knew about nutrition. I started to listen to my body and only my body 100% of the time. I really had no choice. That was the first time in my life I ever did that. It's not that I never listened to my body before; if I was thirsty I would drink water. Duh! But until that point I was always operating within the framework of some dietary dogma I created for myself. It was quite something to let go of all that mental garbage, and learn to actually trust myself. To trust that my body knew exactly what it needed. Everything that went into my mouth was judged, not based on what I read was "good" or "bad", but how it reacted in my body and what my body was craving. Since I made that change, it's been a slow, but steady healing process. All of my health problems have vastly improved. I'm hardly in a state of robust health, but I'm no longer on a downward spiral of disease. Not quite a fairy tale ending. My guess is it will take at least as long to regain my health as it did to lose it.

At one point, I thought I knew a lot about nutrition. I knew what caused disease and what created health. I fanatically pursued those practices for many years in an extremist fashion. And then life kicked me in the nuts. If there is one thing I do know, it's that no food or macronutrient is inherently good or bad. The "goodness" or "badness" of any food can only be determined in relationship to the body of the person that is consuming that food. Dietary rules are static, the body is not. Health has nothing to do with the amount of "good" foods you consume and the amount of "bad" foods you avoid; it has everything to do with how your body uses those foods, which is based on a long list of variables entirely unique to you. Give me any "good" food or any "healthy" habit, and I'll give you a protocol to ruin your health with it. That includes vegetables, water, grass-fed organic animal products, raw butter from Jersey cows, exercise, fasting, or a low-carb paleo diet.

Dental health is one area where the "there are no inherently good or bad foods" holds true. At one time I had a list of foods that I thought were good for my teeth:
– Cod liver oil, skate liver oil
– Liver
– Cultured milk
– Cheese
– Butter, butter oil
– Bone marrow

– Bone broth/stock
– Fish stock
– Kelp and other sea veggies
– Vegetable juice
– Molasses
– Fish eggs (look for discarded carcasses at fish markets)
– Raw cream
– Mustard and tomalley (innards of crab and lobster)
– Animal glands
– Brains
– Intestines
– Blood
– Fish (raw or fermented), especially eyes and head
– Oysters and clams (raw)
– Raw milk
– Supplements
- Ca, Mg
- Clays
- Si, S, Mn, Cu, Zn, B (mixed forms like chelates) (3-6 mg/day)
- Vit-C

And things that I thought were "bad" for my teeth:
– Unsoaked, unsprouted grains, nuts, and seeds
– Sugar, fruit

I adhered to this list pretty religiously, eating huge amounts of grass-fed raw butter, butter oil, skate liver oil, organ meats, bone marrow, fish head stock, and high-mineral foods and supplements. I also avoided nearly all fruit, processed foods, and grains. I binged on nuts occasionally (it was an allowed food).

The result? My teeth stopped getting worse, but never really healed. And when I did eat fruit, say three oranges, my teeth would hurt! I should have had teeth of steel but instead they hurt when I ate a couple pieces of fruit! Another factor was that my sleep was so fucked up that I was grinding my teeth every night.

It's not that those foods aren't important for the teeth, but only in context with the individual's body. My teeth are feeling much better now, even with all the evil sugar in fruit and ice cream and with eating starch with every meal.

Bob

I started to notice I was chubby in like 2nd or 3rd grade. It always bothered me. Everyone always told me I would grow out of it but I didn't believe them. It got even worse when I noticed deep purple stretch marks. I had really big growth spurts, and I guess I would attribute that to my bilateral osgood schlatters disease I was diagnosed with. You know, the swollen knee cap deal. My mother was/is big, and I knew I took after her side of the family more so that didn't sit with me well either. Every year I would say to myself that I would exercise and lose the weight. I don't remember thinking about food much when I was younger. But I never did the exercises, instead I would be on the computer or watch TV. Computer games can seriously suck you in, and I still think they're awesome haha, if only I had time to play them!

Anyhow, at about age 16 I started to read a lot more about nutrition and stuff on the internet. I don't remember what caused this, but it probably had something to do with me looking up my mom's health problems or something. And I'm sure it had plenty to do with tired of being self-conscious, lack of girls, etc…To make a long story short with the beginning of that, I started to read food labels, avoided things with a thousand ingredients, stayed away from "empty calories" such as pop and stuff. This was a slow evolution that took place, but I always went back to reading and developing more of what I thought was the right way. The longer I read, the further I was digging myself into a hole.

I did lose weight, and it was awesome. I walked a lot more, drank crap loads of water, but also there was a dark side of being a teenager. I drank a lot of alcohol when I wasn't busy reading or eating things I thought were healthy. Growing up I didn't have much guidance so I was doing whatever I wanted. For a few years I had ups and downs with achieving that healthy look I've always wanted. Depression, drinking heavily on the weekends, bouts of failure where I'd eat whatever I wanted like whole bags of chicken nuggets. I don't remember when I started to delve into low carbing and paleo to be honest. I can for certain say that I deprived myself of things I really needed at my most important stages of development. Not getting enough calories, and drinking on top of it.

Wowzer…I would eat tuna, and chicken, and tons of green vegetables a lot of the time to "fill" me up. I'm almost six foot six and in retrospect I'm a damn fool for never considering that maybe the foods I was eating wasn't giving me enough energy. There's so much to say…I apologize as I always do for being "all over the place".

Basically, at one point, I had really bad acne (runs in the family) my hair was falling out pretty easy and it was already receded, and I felt like shit. I seriously would think about suicide. I think probably my adrenal glands giving me energy was the only thing that would pull me out of my slumps and get me motivated to be stricter and to read and learn more. During all of these years of trying different stuff (of which I would also try to tell other people what they should and shouldn't do IDIOT) I never attained a six pack, or was muscular and lean like I wanted. I was most muscular when I wasn't reading and was too busy with other things to think about my weight. I had big calves and was pretty strong too before I started this weird diet shit. I lost my calves, I probably stunted my growth, screwed with my puberty, the works.

One day I said to myself, if you're going to be bald, then you better get into shape. Call me shallow, or too self-conscious, but I seriously couldn't stand to live with myself being that fat bald guy with fucking pimples. So more reading I did, more exercise, the stricter I became. I ran across Sean Croxton, Mark Sission, Kurt Harris, a bunch of dudes, and was pretty much low carbing, whole foods, paleo whatever you wanna call it-ing. I lost a lot of weight, the most I ever have. I was really doing it this time, going all the way. I pulled myself together, started working, etc…

My acne would flair up, then I would be strict about avoiding grains and dairy, it would get better, I would give in, blah blah blah, a vicious cycle. Never attained a body that I wanted though. I lost too much weight too fast, my skin is still very loose as I'm typing this. I lost a lot of muscle mass, I guess I was, somewhat am a skinny fat person.

I started a very strenuous job, it broke me out really bad, I was almost passing out doing my work. I at one point went super low carb to try to really turn into a fat burner and fix my energy problems. Didn't work. I think injuries were healing pretty slow too. Bruises, cuts and what not. Eventually I knew I had to increase my carbohydrates. I would do sweet potatoes at night, or regular potatoes but this still wasn't enough. I've known about Matt Stone for a good while, and had heard his interview with Sean Croxton pretty far back I think. My memory I guess is a piece of shit, because I can't even remember right now what led me to start reading this blog and seriously considering a different approach. It's just the time of day for me I think…I'm all foggy I really need to eat lol, and when I do, it's going to be epic. As it has been now for a couple months-ish.

I wanna say my hair isn't falling out anymore, but I could be wrong. Definitely gaining weight. Doing some serious smashing. Bowel movements are much better, food digests much better, hardly ever get light headed anymore. I also think since I have started to become conscious of diluting my bodies salts/sugars, I have less charlie horse issues as well. Food sensitivities have gone WAY down. I haven't been doing this for that long but seriously, the higher my temperature, it's like nothing gives me IBS. High gluten flour pizza's, two of them at one sitting a couple of times, haven't given me any problems. Juice, a whole tub of ice cream at one point, I haven't had those crazy cramps and the urge to you know what from all this "shit" I've been eating. It's incredible, I'm going to keep doing it and have what I want. When I make more money I'll look into mineral supplementation for sure.

I missed a thousand points, and could say a billion more things, but the bottom line is, for a long time I thought I knew what I was doing and I was dead wrong. I hope I didn't hurt anybody by giving them the wrong advice. And the paleolithic movement definitely has some really positive perspectives don't get me wrong. I am thankful that I am still alive and my journey has definitely been quite the learning experience.

Stephon

I have been following Paleo/ Primal style eating since May '10 and initially as others have stated I felt great energy wise, and went from 164 lbs to 152 lbs in a month's time with full 6 pack abs! I always figured I was carb sensitive so the results only convinced me more… fast forward to Sept 2011 and I have developed a "Full Blown" phobia of carbs, wouldn't even eat a piece of cake for my daughter's birthday, or the cheesecake (which I used to love) for my own birthday? I have suffered severe Insomnia and the cold hands, and at night sometimes the sweats are ridiculous waking up to use the bathroom several times even though I stop drinking fluids at 3 or 4 P.M.? Not even going to get me started on my SEX DRIVE! Not to get too personal but I used to get some crazy erections and now I'm like huh?

Yesterday I was having dinner with a friend and it was about 73 degrees outside in Orlando and suddenly I became cold. I looked at my hands and my fingernails were a bluish color, showed my friend and they were like wtf? I blew it off but am a bit concerned now. I'm having a beer as I type this because I'm soo stressed out and feeling extremely guilty about drinking the beer? My roommate says I have become a completely different person, just irritable and short fused. He eats drinks and I watch with envy! Too worried about regaining my weight which was initially 186lbs @ 5'5'? . Everyone tells me that all the meat and fat can't be healthy without carbs and as much as I want to have carbs on a consistent basis, I'm seriously struggling too concerned with losing what I seemingly have achieved with this lifestyle.

Not sure rather or not I mentioned that I fast daily too! I don't really know where to start to be honest but I know something has to give and so far the only thing that has given has been my sanity as well as my relationship with food. I've always loved carbs and on the one day that I do eat them I go crazy and want nothing but carbs, and sweets. I enjoy working out and being active but don't want to be obsessing over whether I will regain all the weight back I have previously lost.

My alcohol tolerance has went as well, not that I'm big on drinking but I enjoy a few drinks on the weekend. Seriously I seem to always have to wear a hoody even in my apt because I feel cold most the time.

Nuka

Currently I am a 33 year old female, been always working out a lot and very active, Crossfit since 2007. Since late teens I've paid attention to what I eat due to my sports hobbies.

First I ate like a decade of low fat including aspartame and all that shit, light cheese and stuff. Tons of quark, cottage cheese, tuna. Tho I DO love them, or I WOULD if I'd still eat those.

Then started going low carb and that went well, shed some body% but only after some years on low carb. Was always normal, athletic size/build. Got to know paleo and went fully paleo in 01/2010. Before I was quite low carb but still are some dairy. I haven't been eating grains in years really.
Anyway, I was in optimal shape and condition when going paleo. First it seemed to make things even better; I shed some more body% ending up at 15% which was pretty lean for me (was 17% for years). When going paleo I also read Nora Gedgaudas's book *Primal Body, Primal Mind*. She totally convinced me that ALL carb is bad and you want to minimise insulin. So I quit eating fruit, tubers and roots and berries. Two months after (four months on paleo) things started to accumulate.

First I rapidly lost 3-4 kgs when I had diarrhea for a month. Then I started gaining FAST. I was also so, so tired, worn out, didn't recover from exercise, was freezing cold all the time, my period was absent, no sex drive, anxiety attacks (or something like that, never saw anyone about these but bursts or anger or despair) and a dozen other symptoms. Because I was gaining weight fast my solution was to eat even LESS carbs and exercise MORE! Winner.

My cortisol went sky high and I went on eating low carb for 1.5 years still after things were accumulating. My weight stayed at 13 kg higher than I'd been for years before and it still is. In 03/2011 I got myself a subclinical hypothyroidism diagnosis and started T4. First it helped a little but not for long. I also got terrible joint pain.

Then finally at the end of 08/2011 things started to unravel and I had my RT3 tested. It was super high compared to my T3. I started T3 only meds in 09/2011 and since then my symptoms have all resolved. All except weight gain, but I'm determined to get back into my own size whatever it takes. Since I believe that what caused high RT3 originally was ketogenic diet plus excessive exercise = stress, I think I should be able to get off meds little by little. I got my recent labs last week and they looked good: TSH 0,006, T4 5,2 and T3 4,0. Hb 140 and ferritin 81 (5-100).

Oh yes, about the diet; I still eat "paleo" ie. no grains, no dairy, no sugar, no legumes and I stick to it like 95%, sometimes a little cheese. But after reading stuff by Paul Jaminet I added safe starches aka rice to my diet two months ago. I've felt good. Still, I'm SO looking forward to lose some weight. Any ideas? ;-D

And I was one of those that once they start something they'll stick to it to stupidity… I followed paleo to a T, really. Low carb paleo, needless to mention. A bit obsessive mind as I am. :-) Luckily I've been able to exercise the whole time (or actually I just wouldn't give it up despite how wrecked I was at a time because it's so important for me) and I'm never sick.

Anyway, almost everything has improved. Now just trying to figure out what to do about the weight... Been cutting down fat consumption now that I eat more carbs.
Long story, sorry for that! Hope the info's useful for someone :-) **YIKES!!!! Haha**

Jared Bond

First, my thoughts on Paleo. I think we agree that the heart of Paleo is in a good place. Modern society has been blindsided by obesity and disease, and we don't really know why. Many get the feeling our diet is somehow deficient, and I think most of us here still believe that. The health of primitive humans (or even those in more recent history) seems like it was better, so it makes sense to try and figure out what they did right and we did wrong. I'm inclined to think people do get more of the stuff we need doing Paleo— vitamins, minerals, and maybe even fiber. But waiting for people who want to investigate this idea are all sorts of traps: the low-carb trap, the no-sugar trap, the low-calorie trap, the raw trap, the anti-nutrient trap, the "fat's not bad so now it's the best thing ever" trap... these are the real dangers, specifically for those who are already sick.

I truly empathize with people getting freaked out by the availability of food items that were almost certainly not available to our ancestors. Can any of us seriously imagine going our entire lives without soda, milkshakes, or candy bars? Or even the wide array of fruit we have these days? And yet, our ancestors seemed to have done just fine without it. When I started thinking about changing my diet, I didn't see why I should so desperately need something that our species didn't for millions of years (or even just hundreds of years). And so at the very least, I didn't think it would be harmful to completely abstain from such things. I thought maybe I needed to toughen up.

And probably nothing will convince people that this is not the way to go unless they really try it for themselves. Sure, we could expect that a period of adjustment would be necessary. But I did very low carb for over a year, and no fructose for 3 months, and it never felt right. My "enzymes" didn't adjust. I felt deprived, was very gaunt, got gout on two occasions, spent way too much time and energy worrying about food, and had chronically loose stools which I've never had before or since. (I couldn't even believe it was gout at the time, because I'm not fat or middle-aged.) This went on way longer than it should have, and it was for two reasons: my psychological circumstances, and the seemingly overwhelming scientific support and testimony. It's a nightmare to think of how long I may have continued my diet if it weren't for Matt Stone.

I know most people are not as extreme as I was. It's good to know that not all Paleos are low-carb. But my hope for this book is that it helps people retain the ability to listen to their body despite everything they think or have read.

Still, my story might be relevant because all low-carbers are in some sense Paleo. The biggest supporting argument for low-carb is how you simply cannot get a lot of carbs without agriculture, cooking, and widespread trade (at least for people of European ancestry). I don't think the stuff about fructose and insulin would really sound plausible if it weren't for this background.

People can argue that we can't really know what pre-humans did, but here's the thing– I was convinced that, at least at some point in our history, pre-humans were carnivorous. It seemed that at some point our hominid lineage would be smart enough to spread all over the world, but not smart enough to cook or grow food; and so the only significant thing around was meat. Also, we appeared to be adapted to survive through repeated ice-ages. Again, at the very least, I did not think it could possibly be harmful to eat a diet that we were at some point biologically adapted for. (Our small appendix was one of the things that convinced me.)

Yes, it seems really sick to me today, (and did even then), but here's the other reason why I went to a mostly meat diet: Meat was being touted by low-carb authors as the perfect food. They said that fat is the body's preferred fuel– that's why it stores its energy as fat. They said we need a lot of protein, and the body would make whatever glucose it needed from that, keeping it at a stable level, instead of the dreaded spikes. As Michael Eades liked to say, "There is no such thing as a necessary carbohydrate!" Also, meat had all the vitamins and minerals in their most digestible form, and no anti-nutrients. One example that really impacted me was how Stefansson said that a person could live for years in perfect health on pemmican alone.

I decided that to get on the fast track to "healing", or at least shock my body into the right direction, it was easiest just to eliminate pretty much all plant foods entirely. I became afraid of everything besides meat, even milk with its opiod-like casein. My influences were Gary Taubes, Mike Eades, Barry Groves, Tom Naughton, and Natasha Campbell-McBride and the whole GAPS theory, Lierre Keith, Nora Gedgaudas, Aajonus Vonderplanitz, the "Fiber Menace" guy, Ron Schmid, some lady from Poland, William Dufty's "Sugar Blues", and the WAPF. Between all of them, their techniques seemed to be able to help or cure every disease under the sun (even MS, as noted by Barry Groves). And eliminating carbs, fiber, and antinutrients seemed to be the common thread. So it seemed my best bet would be to eliminate all of them. (I had a vague idea that maybe I had blood sugar issues, or perhaps some other unidentifiable cause for chronic fatigue.) Assurances that I would be getting enough calories and be able to digest that much protein and fat were built on scanty evidence, but people who are desperate don't wait around to investigate. (Sadly, in the end, this probably WAS the easiest way for me to find out whether or not those assurances were true.)

I expect that most people instinctively would not come to such an extreme conclusion. But I was desperate, and if one takes the theories behind low-carb to their literal implications, desperation may very well push you until you reach this extreme. It's ridiculous, but this is the low-carb trap. Most people will just lightly do low-carb (and live with constant guilt), but if you truly believe that insulin and sugars are the bane of human biology, then you have to conclude that this is the ideal diet– even if you personally find it impossible to follow.

As silly as it was, I really, really thought it was the truth, because the concurrence of all the science and books just seemed unshakable. (–even DESPITE how psychologically messed up it was to think that "healthy" and "ideal" calls for an all-out animal bloodbath. I REALLY regret trying to incorporate that idea into my entire worldview.) What really caught my attention about Matt Stone is that he had read ALL of them, and still had the ability to say no to the whole thing. I honestly didn't think that was possible. I thought insulin separated the men from the boys. Even the mainstream is tending against carbs and fructose these days, so I saw that as confirmation of low-carb's validity. And the fact that people DO lose weight on it.

Also, the follower enthusiasm of any diet can really be misleading. I thought low-carb was working out great for everyone who did it, because all I read were good comments. I was sincerely shocked when Matt Stone did a post on Tom

Naughton's blog, and then everyone's negative stories came out of the woodwork, seemingly out of nowhere. I was also shocked when I made a thread on "Raw Paleo Forum" with the headline "Insulin spikes do NOT cause insulin resistance??" (http://www.rawpaleodietforum.com/hot-topics/insulin-spikes-do-not-cause-insulin-resistance/), and significant figures on the site were coming out and saying how they don't think carbs are harmful and so on.

Now, I wasn't quite as extreme as some of those people, but they were really the example in my mind of how people were actually DOING the diet I was advocating, and appeared to be doing well. I had assumed they were all in agreement, and that this was the ideal diet for everyone. But that turned out to be my own delusion! Also what was interesting about that thread—I had posted it in the "Carnivorous / Zero Carb Approach" section, precisely because I wanted it to reach people like me, who would only be browsing that section of the forum. That subject line would have gotten my attention. But people got mad over it. Some had the attitude of "What are you doing here?", and just wanted me to leave. Eventually, a moderator moved it to the "Hot Topics" section, a place where I never would have looked. It goes to show how some people really don't want to learn more, but only want a support group to encourage them to continue doing their odd or strenuous activities. It reminded me a little of online anorexia support groups.

Lastly, it's always more convincing when there's a conspiracy element attached to anything. Most people will at least believe that corporations and institutions will put profits before the people. The shock of learning that some aspect of mainstream health is wrong can too easily lead us to champion the opposite, almost as an act of revenge, or defiance. And of course, with all the other conspiracy stuff going on out there, one can begin to doubt the very fundamentals of their upbringing and society. I can't really say much about this other than, don't lose your head. And try not to fall for a story just because it's sensational. Through all this, I've learned that we just can't know nearly as much as we think we can from reading books and listening to "experts". Even with competent scientists, the complexities of biology and chemistry usually cannot be reduced to such simplicity. We have complex tastes and particularities for a reason. And everyone's unique. Perhaps we can't always trust our intuition and feelings, and occasionally need to reform ourselves based on intellectual theory, but I would never mistrust my feelings and common tradition that much again. This now common view of sugar (or even carbs) as an addictive "drug" instead of the easiest to use energy really makes me sad, as it is probably making life unnecessarily harder for a lot of people.

Anonymous

I got onto the Paleo bandwagon after reading Mark Sisson's *Primal Blueprint* in February 2010. My motivation: getting that ripped and muscular body that so many of the success testimonials had posted on MarksDailyApple. I think this is an important detail. Without this motivation, I probably would not have been able to mobilize the discipline with which I embarked on this diet journey.

I remember the feel of this diet. It was a funny feeling. It felt a bit like having drunk way too much water in order to kill your thirst. I never felt satisfied despite just having eaten a salad, some fruit, and tons of eggs. I read on a forum that what I experienced was the carb flu and that it would pass. After about three weeks, I had dinner with my husband. He had not yet become used to my new dietary regime (dictatorship would be a more appropriate term) and had prepared too little meat. I had to eat the potatoes that he had cooked because there was not enough primal-approved food around to get satisfied. Boy, I felt so elated. It was like being on drugs. Better than chocolate. It should have taught me something but I was much too stubborn to listen.

The next day I was back on track. I started to feel better then. I noticed some startling improvements. The eczema in my face started to vanish. I felt hot the whole time (I was able to start the day with a cold shower). My sleep was profound and refreshing. It was great. And I started to lose weight. The right kind of weight. My pants started to fit again.

Then I began a lifting routine. 5x5. It was strenuous but I liked the training schedule because the sessions were quite short. I also started sprinting as suggested in the *Primal Blueprint*. In late April, my weight loss stalled. I had lost 10 pounds since I had started in late February which was amazing. Still, I wanted to lose more so I started IFing, too. Just one day every two weeks (but without catching up on the calories). The funny feeling from the beginning returned. I started to feel sick more and more frequently. The eczema came back.

I have to be doing something wrong, I thought. I bought some keto sticks and restricted my carb intake even further to attain that fabled state of ketosis which would finally solve my weight problems - at least that was the impression I was under after reading the respective chapter again and again. I was able to achieve a state of mild ketosis every couple of days. Yet, instead of feeling better I started to feel worse. What's more: I felt guilty.

See, I didn't have any problems combining the Paleo diet with my lifestyle. I had eggs, salad and fruit in the morning, some meat, vegetables for lunch and dinner coupled with lots of butter. As long as I did not go to a vegan restaurant I would find something on the menu at every place where I would meet my friends. The social aspect of the diet was not the problem. I got obsessed though with the moral implications of this lifestyle. All those animal lives I was taking just to satisfy my vanity. I made sure that I bought the best organic, grass-fed blah blah you can find in an urban agglomeration but the fact that I could afford this stuff somehow made it even worse. Shouldn't every human being be entitled to good health? I wondered. I started thinking about the ethical aspects of agriculture. There are some big holes in veganism if you look at it from the point of view of ideology but was my ideology better? Lierre Keith had some convincing arguments but did they add up? I remember spending whole evenings doing calculations of meat needed to feed a certain group of people Paleo style. How much land you would need to raise the necessary cattle on. How much land was available - and recognizing that this was in no way a sustainable way to feed myself, not to mention the world population.

Still, I persisted. (I am still astonished when I think of the discipline with which I ate and exercised - I have never been able to muster up that kind of commitment before or after that episode in my life. I was a zealot.)

In late May, I experienced a sharp pain in my stomach one day after breakfast. The pain continued until late in the afternoon. I couldn't eat because it hurt so much. I went to see the doctor the next day. She told me that I had a condition called gastroparesis and that I should take medication against it. It would go away. I started taking the pills. The pain did go away. My hunger returned and it was stronger than ever. I drank coconut oil tea because I thought that that would fill me up and provide enough calories. (I regularly consumed 3,000 to 4,000 calories per day at the time drinking like whole cups of cream and did not gain weight by the way. It was an interesting experiment in that it put the calories make you fat theory to rest - at least for me.) The only thing I got from it was diarrhea. It was so bad that I had to stay home from work one day.

I got desperate. My weight stalled, my health problems returned, I couldn't sleep. Then, one day in June, I had to go on a business trip. The business trips were the only time when I had problems feeding myself. I had resorted to eating lots of dark chocolate on these trips because that was the only Paleo-approved food available at train stations. Now I was sitting on this train and feeling worse than ever. It was my stomach again. It felt as if somebody was poking me with a dagger.

I arrived at my destination. The meeting with my colleagues was still some hours away so I decided to go to a restaurant and have lunch. The waiter took my order - some steak as always. I was a bit unsure how I would be able to gag it down with my stomach hurting like it was. The waiter brought a bread basket. I eyed the bread and something inside me clicked. I had a slice. And another. And then suddenly the pain went away. I ate the bread, the steak and the side of potatoes with relish. It was great. I have never experienced something like this in my entire life. Killing pain by eating food.

I discovered 180DegreeHealth by searching gastroparesis on the paleo forums. In many respects it has been a god-send. I started to eat the food. I gained the 10 pounds I had lost and then another 20. Must be my body's revenge on me. I had a hard time feeling satiated. I would eat potatoes, 2 pounds with butter and steak and veggies and still feel hungry. I rrarfed repeatedly. **(RRARF is a somewhat comical acronym I created referring to my program for raising metabolism – it stands for Rehabilitative Rest and Aggressive Refeeding. Because you eat a lot, the name "RRARF" reminded me** of the sound of vomiting. I'm weird I know. Shut up. I cut yo face man!)

My stint at paleo ended almost 17 months ago. I still have my health problems, the eczema, the erratic sleeping patterns, the headaches, but I have finally come to terms with my weight. Well sort of. I have my bad days but I can cope with them. I am still latently hypothyroid and I have little testosterone. My cholesterol is not too good either. My endocrinologist thinks it would be a good idea if I lost some fat (he told me that the fat cells convert testosterone to estrogen). I took up weight lifting again last November but somehow I have lost my zest for it. My knees hurt when I do it or I get sick. And I am not too sure that I am making any progress from it in the health department. I also have some other symptoms of low testosterone: I regularly break into a sweat even when the rest of my body feels cold, I don't sleep well. My libido is going strong (hooray one thing is still working properly) but that is about it.

To sum my experience up: Paleo was an interesting experiment which has taught me a lot about how flawed much of the current ideologies in nutrition are, but I paid a huge price for it. To anyone who reads this and considers Paleo - don't do it. It can seriously f*** you up.

Anonymous

I discovered your website very recently and it's been interesting to go through the posts and comments! For a long time I thought there was not one soul against or even criticizing the paleo movement. I certainly wasn't! I trusted it like my grandmother despite the signals my body was trying to send me. Here's my story.

I've been scared of carbs since 2004. That was when I first tried Atkins and lost a bunch of weight. Since then I've tried many other things but deep down I've always thought that I must avoid carbs at any cost; even when I was training five hours a day, six days a week. (Yeah!) That was in 2009 and the lowest point in my life.

That extreme madness lasted for about two months until I finally realized that if I would continue any longer, I would die. I rather risked getting fat (the worst sin of all) than check into a mental hospital. So I started training a lot less (maybe just an hour or two every day), I slept more and had a big breakfast every day: toast, cheese, coffee, yoghurt and fruit. Then I took some time off and biked over to have a big lunch (oh, I loved it): loads of whatever was available and a portion of chocolate mousse every day. I wasn't over-stuffed but I was feeling so so satisfied. In the evening I had whatever I fancied. The weight just fell off and I felt fantastic.

I don't know why but after a while (around 2009) I started paleo. I had heard so many good things about it. I have never been happy with what I have so I thought maybe I could finally lose the last 10lbs and get a six pack. Since then I've been on and off paleo; I've always done my best but was never able to be perfect so blamed myself for being a loser and tried even harder.

I was looking at all those PBP **(Primal Blueprint)** success stories and fantasizing about my own success but it never came. I was carbophobic and scared of food. Occasionally I was eating only meat, nothing else. That made me feel really really s**t but I thought it was what the Eskimos did so it must be really great. (Although I was still a little guilty because I did cook my food and didn't eat it raw. Now this just makes me laugh, what a moron I was.)

For me the worst was when everyone kept saying how this paleo thing is the answer to everything; if you just stick with it, all your problems, including cancer, all autoimmune diseases and allergies just vanish and you'll live forever. Not that I ever had any of those anyway but I started imagining that I was insulin and leptin resistant and so on. (Oh god.)

The thing is, when I was a kid, I was never allergic to anything. I ate whatever I was given and that was just fine. All my problems appeared when I started to "improve" my diet. That was maybe 17 years ago (I'm 31 now).

What troubles me is that since people learn about paleo, they start treating their bodies like they are really sensitive and need extra enzymes, probiotics and careful timing to be able to handle a potato. *Wouldn't evolution make sure that we are equipped to handle a large variety of foods - even relatively modern varieties?*

I've also been wondering *why it would be better for me to eat loads of sweet potatoes and coconut (especially processed coconut cream) that so many generations before me (my own ancestors) have not even seen - just because paleolithic people may have eaten that way somewhere on the other side of the world.*

I've started to question how people (everyone who starts paleo suddenly becomes a nutrition expert) talk about lectins and anti-nutrients and stuff. I'm sorry but how do they know? *Like really know?* They don't! They've read it somewhere and then they walk around pretending like they know everything. Okay, I was guilty of this too.

See, when I learned about paleo I (too) started blogging about it. I also wrote a couple of articles about it (I'm a journalist) and organized a paleo seminar. I can see how people can make money out of it. I did.

What I've realized is that it is more important to me to relax, to love and enjoy life and to be able to go to a friend's place and tell them *yes, I will eat whatever you lovingly cook me.* I no longer like the idea of someone else telling me what to eat. How do they know? They don't live in my body! **(Um, we are going to need some double-blind, peer-reviewed studies to show us that this won't make you drop dead of a heart attack at 48!!!)**

Paleo also always left me feeling deprived - although this is something that I denied. *Why do we desperately want carbs if they are meant to be so bad for us?*

Why did I fall into that paleo trap?

What did paleo do for me? It did make me respect the quality of food and source organic, local stuff. It made me fearless of fat - maybe too much so because I gained a lot of weight. It made me part of this tribe and I got to know loads of new people. People who will probably be shocked when I tell them I'm back to eating porridge with jam, baked potatoes, fabulous bread and cheese, amazing yoghurt, pizza, tacos, peanut butter and bananas. I still spend a small fortune on food because for me quality is the key and I have no plans to start stuffing myself with processed crap. But I do want to enjoy whatever there is. Hell yeah, it's my life!

When I look back, I cannot believe I based my diet - no, my whole life - on what cavemen may have eaten and how they may have lived. That is ridiculous.

It's only been about a week but I feel like a (newborn) queen. I feel like by cheeks are getting a healthy glow from just the pure pleasure of feeling free to feed myself whatever I want. No quilt, no nonsense. And all that time I have left when I no longer have to spend my time in front of the computer checking out the latest paleo news; *which one is worse this week, glucose or fructose?*

Thank you Matt Stone.

Anonymous

After the birth of my second child, I had about 15lbs I just couldn't lose. First I tried WW, then low carb, then high fat, finally paleo. Throughout this time (2 years). I'd lose a few pounds then regain. Oh and I would alternate between running every day for an hour and then doing nothing because I was so freakin tired. Anyways, paleo seemed great at first because I could eat carbs again (cue harps and angels). Imagine....apples and squash.... but not too much. And dates and more spaghetti squash (which tastes nothing like spaghetti by the way).. oh but just 1/2 cup. Wait but I want some bean soup! Beans aren't allowed....um but you can pick them right? Uh yeah but not 100,000 years ago. But the obesity problem is only like 80 years old. Shut up and eat your coconut flour pancakes!! How did people make coconut flour pancakes 100,000 years ago? (cue crickets). Well needless to say, a few weeks ago, I threw in the towel. I had lost like 5 lbs, was always cold and moody and just hated food- oh except for chocolate. Since dark chocolate is apparently ok in moderation according to some paleo preachers, I indulged in a bar every few days. Hey that's moderation compared to every day, right?

Since I had only skimmed 180 Degree Health and didn't have time to read in depth (due to all of my hunting, gathering and moving slowly), I took what I knew and dove in. First, 3 meals a day. Boy was I happy to have a pancake or oats or (gasp) toast!! After going through 5 dozen eggs/week on paleo or LC, I was so glad to not have to choke down yet another yolk if I didn't want to. Lunchtime... dare I have a sandwich? A bowl of split pea soup? Why yes I shall. How about dinner... rice and veggies WITHOUT 3 pounds of beef?!? Right here please. And that chocolate or ice cream? In the afternoon please after I finished a short workout on the elliptical or a little rebounding- yes I have one and it's awesome and fun!

Results? Couple pounds lost, no food obsessing, much better sleep (as in, hitting the pillow by 10pm, asleep by 10:10 and up by 7 feeling refreshed. I even managed to take a two hour nap with my kids one day. Totally unthinkable a few months ago). Another plus; since I don't have to eat meat at every meal (and really how sustainable is that) our grocery bill has decreased. Just a nice bonus. Oh and my hubby and kids think mom was replaced by some angel who will cook anything they are hungry for without inquiring about our ancestral connection (or lack thereof) to the requested food. I'm pretty sure I have more friends now too that I'm not preaching about how evil popcorn is. It's just a snack- sheesh!!

Anonymous

Dear Matt Stone,

As I read your fake Paleo fail story **(I wrote a generic Paleo story on my blog once)** it was like I was reading my own, but without a happy ending. Here is my story: I have never been overweight; I am a 6ft tall woman and I weigh between 145-150 lbs. I sought out a Paleo diet because I thought it would cure my health issues. In August of 2010 I had a second trimester miscarriage after suffering through a 3+ months of pregnancy and being terribly ill for most of it (sinusitis, followed by antibiotics followed by severe yeast infection). Even after the miscarriage, the yeast infection never went away despite all the remedies, natural and not, so in October 2010 I found this diet to try to control the candida and help with my PCOS, insulin resistance, and chronic fatigue. It was so extreme (even beyond Paleo!) I was only able to do it for four months eating only about 15-20 net carb grams a day. My skin improved and I lost a bunch of weight I didn't need to lose, but that is basically the extent of the effects.

In February 2011 I switched to GAPS/ Paleo but stayed low carb getting around 50 grams of carb a day as every time I tried to add carby veg I would have severe yeast flareups. From everything I read in the Primal/Paleo camp, I didn't need the carby veg and much fruit anyway. Fructose especially was bad so the only fruit I would eat was lemons, berries, and green apples and only once or twice a week. At this time I was only eating two or three times a day at most and I started getting eczema from eating dairy which I ended up cutting out entirely (aside from Ghee) in September. In June my periods started to go whacky, I started to get VERY tender breasts for a week before my period (something that I never had before), I started to put on weight on my belly and thighs, became very depressed, struggled with insomnia, frequent constipation and started to have anxiety issues. Which leads us to now: I now have zero sex drive which my husband and I are very unhappy about.

I have obviously been stressing my adrenals and I need to fix this. I desperately want to be healthy and I am tired of being led down so many wrong roads. I am so afraid to add more carbs to my diet for fear of the yeast beast and having been indoctrinated by Bee and the Paleo camp that too many carbs are bad. I am afraid of having setbacks on GAPS by trying to add in too many foods too fast. During the last few days I am trying to eat more and get more sleep. I have been supplementing with magnesium oil, zinc, B complex, anything I can find to support my adrenals. I honestly have no idea what to do next. It is certainly too early to say whether or not your plan will work but I need to try something.

Anonymous

Hello Matt! First let me say thank you for your website and free information. It truly is a blessing. I discovered you through East West Healing, so thanks to them as well. Anyway this terribly written letter is about how diets, PALEO IN PARTICULAR made me feel like crap! In fact over the past ten years my best times were when I was "off the wagon" so to speak!

Although I have experimented in dieting since age 15. I had certification through NTA for holistic nutrition and WITS for personal training. I have spent thousands upon thousands of dollars on nutrition books and supplements. I have spent so much time preparing strange concoctions from raw food smoothies made from lettuce to kombucha. I truly have tried every diet!

I was a chubby kid from about 12 years old and I just wanted to be "normal." Dieting, as you know, just makes you more abnormal. People made fun of me, friends and family didn't understand and I was miserable. This went on for years. I am 26 now and just starting to get my health back via some of yours and Dr. Peat's ideas.

I think the thing that made me hit rock bottom was the paleo diet. Even though I had dabbled in raw veganism and lacto-ovo vegetarianism, paleo crashed me hard. I think probably due to the severe carb restriction. I suffered headaches for the first time in my life, low sex drive (i'm 26 yrs old male), cold hands and feet, lack of energy and probably depression, though it wasn't diagnosed. Basically I felt like crap.

Others who I persuaded to try these diets have had similar results. My only intention here is to hopefully give someone out there hope that they can stop the vicious cycle of yo - yo dieting that I wasted so much time on. I have probably missed out on hundreds of celebrations with friends and family needlessly. Sitting in my chair with a bowl of fruit in front of me and nothing else. Jealous of everyone who seemed to be able to eat whatever they want without consequences. What a way to live one's teens and twenties!!!

My quest is not without its rewards though. I have learned so many interesting things about chemistry and biology. I have had some great experiences helping others lose weight and feel better with just minor lifestyle changes. I just seem to lack the moderation to follow my own simple advice sometimes.

I am here to tell you that in the few weeks that I have been following your advice I seem to have a clarity that I lacked before. I can see how I was starving my body and brain of energy by my sugar phobia. Thank goodness I somehow managed to keep an open mind about food enough to hear what you and others like you have to say.

And yes my sex drive came roaring back, my sleep is deeper, my energy at work is higher and most importantly my usual optimistic outlook on life came back! Thank you thank you thank you!

Anonymous

So, here is my low carb story...I was not Paleo exactly...I was a self-diagnosed fast-oxidizer, parasympathetic type, also known as a protein type by Mercola,...it was recommended I eat mostly protein, veggies and fats...to stay away from carbs almost entirely, even whole grains. I struggled with this for a long time. I tried desperately to eliminate carbohydrates and mostly did not eat them. I had been diagnosed with Syndrome X, which is high blood pressure and insulin resistance. A doctor had prescribed a blood sugar meter and I got obsessed. I was measuring after every meal and snack I ate...I was beserk. I had no peace. I lived this way for a number of months, perhaps 9 months. I felt good for a while, but what I noticed was that I was not sleeping well, was wired all the time, and had dark circles under my eyes.

When I eventually found 180 Degree Health, I ordered all of Matt's books...in fact, the way I found out about Matt was because I was researching going the Raw Paleo route...and found Matt Stone's work and ordered his package of books...with a sense of courage and optimism I started eating starches again. At the risk of sounding dramatic, I can honestly say it changed my life. I started to chill out again. Eating brown rice felt like this manna from heaven. Red potatoes, grits, sprouted grain bread...OMG! The circles under my eyes went away, I started sleeping more soundly again. I just started to feel human. I stopped measuring my blood sugar. I just wanted to give myself a break, and I have not really returned to doing it.

I know my blood sugar has stabilized though, because of the way I feel. I remember noticing that my sugar obsession was gone just a little bit into the experiment eating carbs again...it's like when I was not eating carbs, sugar seemed massively appealing...no more. My body was just needing carbs and healthy sugar. This is interesting because I had incorporated the belief that when I ate carbs and sugar then I would crash and then I would crave more carbs and sugar...this is a lie. This is absolutely false. 100% not true. Eating carbs again has freed me from senseless food obsessions. I am free. And I am becoming less and less obsessed over time.

I believe in trusting my body. I am learning to add in the common sense, nutrient dense whole foods that nature made and trusting my body about the rest. I believe my nervous system is articulating to me on a minute by minute basis what it needs in every way. I am opening to hear what it is saying and becoming the Health Expert that I had been searching for all along.

Anonymous

Mine is a story of guilt and deprivation. And acid reflux.
I had been on some sort of diet since the age of 12 when my mother, trying to help me lose weight, took me to a diet doctor who gave me large pills he called "amphetamines" and a simple diet plan of 1,000 calories a day. The pills took my appetite away, made me thirsty and very grumpy. But I could ride my bicycle faster than any other kid in my neighborhood! As my heart raced and pounded in my chest, my body quickly shed 30 pounds and for the first time I felt I looked normal. I was happy and it was time to stop the pills and start eating a normal diet again. Uh oh… need I say that within the year I was, somehow, someway, 50 pounds heavier?

This started me on a path of "healthy deprivation" that led me from one diet to the next, including a mostly vegan diet for 20 years. I became cold, my body temperature hovered around 96 degrees. If I had a temperature of 98 or 98.6, it was because I was sick with the flu. My hair thinned out, my teeth got cavities, my nails thinned and hardly grew, I was constantly bloated and filled with gas, but I felt at least lucky that I somehow managed to stay within a somewhat healthy weight, never more than 10 or so pounds too much. Most importantly, I ignored the little voice inside of me that told me I needed more. I needed animal proteins, and I needed them badly, yet my yoga teacher and my professors in college all expounded on the virtues of the low-fat vegetarian diet. Damn the EXPERTS! I kept it up until I was finally convinced by a

Chinese doctor that I must begin at once to eat fish and lamb and other animal proteins. And so I did.

The meat helped me warm up and have better digestion, but still I needed to reduce my weight to something a bit more realistic for my height, so as I decided to jump on the low carbohydrate bandwagon, only to find that I couldn't go too low in carbs because I trembled so badly and fell into what I called a "brain depression". I could stay around 60 -75 grams per day with just a minimal amount of constant shakiness. Based on what the "experts" were saying, I upped my fat intake and lowered my grains and starches even more. I stayed away from grains, fruit, legumes and dairy and eventually developed acid reflux.

Eleven years went by and I couldn't help myself. In fact, no doctor or naturopath could help me either. And the only way I could stop the reflux was to eat nothing but meat and non starchy vegetables which left me a shaking, trembling, depressed, overweight mess of a human being with high blood sugar! My fasting sugars were near 100, but how could that be? I was not eating grains or dairy or fruit or beans!! Something was terribly wrong! I would have days when I could not help myself and I would "accidentally" eat a roll at a restaurant or have a few bites of potato. Then I would suffer with acid reflux, gastritis and an inflamed esophagus, and I would lie in my bed feeling terrible guilt and vowing never to eat another bite of anything that would hurt my body. I reasoned that my occasional indiscretions must be the reason I had higher than normal blood sugar. And I vowed once again: No grains, no fruit, no legumes, no milk or other dairy products, no sugars of any sort… Yet I would still have my weaknesses. And the guilt persisted. Damn the EXPERTS!
I was crying internally for help. My body felt cold on the inside and I had no joy and no desire to move or exercise or go out

for dinner or socialize at all. I couldn't eat, I couldn't drink and I was basically sad and depressed, never mind that I was constantly trembling such that I could barely turn the page of a book.

In 2011, I was fortunate enough to meet Matt Stone and hear him talk about metabolism. It was like magically all the pieces of my "puzzle of deprivation" seemed to come together. I was beside myself with eagerness to learn as much as I could. It felt so right! Needless to say, I began to eat everything and in all the quantities I wanted. I gained some weight as Matt told me I might as I began to heal my metabolism. Mostly, I didn't care; I just wanted to heal. I realized that by my deprivation (basically starving myself of grains and enough carbohydrates) I was digging myself into a deeper and deeper hole that I could not find a way out of. My cold body, my low metabolism was getting worse.

Once I began to eat a wide variety of food again, especially bread and grains and pancakes and quick breads, my digestion began to heal. The first few days were a struggle, both physically and mentally but soon my stomach stopped hurting and everything got better. My hands warmed up and my feet got warmer, too. My joy returned and so did feelings of absolute bliss and peace inside my body. I have learned so much, and most importantly, that my powerful inner voice should never be ignored, just because "experts" (damn them all!) were telling me different! And second, I have learned that no food group is bad; a healthy person should be able to eat all categories of foods including grains! I am so grateful that I have my life and all of my food back, and a much happier belly!

Aaron

Four or five years ago I was a healthy, young, relatively fit individual with no hang-ups or disordered mindsets around food. I ate what I wanted, when I wanted, and didn't worry about it. I had the desire to learn to cook and wanted to incorporate a wider variety of ethnic foods into my palate. I was one of a very small group of my coworkers that would actually go to the Indian, or the Turkish, or the Vietnamese restaurant. But I also didn't stress about dinner. Cottage cheese on toast was a perfectly valid dinner.

I'd been a minor nutrition nerd starting at some point after I got out of college. My go to sources for a while were the Harvard School of Public Health website and NutritionData.com. I felt like these provided decent, albeit basic explanations of nutritional principles. I was first introduced to the concept of low-carb by an article on kuro5hin entitled The Great Modern Glucose Poisoning Epidemic. I didn't act on this information right away but instead just let it set and percolate for a while. I started exploring Blood Sugar 101 and eventually picked up a copy of Gary Taubes' *Good Calories, Bad Calories*.

I'm not a person to withstand cognitive dissonance and I was starting to experience quite a lot of it. I wasn't really in a hurry to give up my breakfast cereal and orange juice habit, but my understanding of modern diseases had shifted drastically. Thanks to Taubes and Blood Sugar 101, I now believed "metabolic syndrome" to be the central disorder and felt that the science pretty solidly established carbohydrates as the sole, direct, causal factor. Eventually I decided to do a few blood sugar tests of my own. I went to Walgreens and bought a glucose meter. That's when it really began.

Had my first tests not shown a fasting of 100mg/dl and a one-hour post prandial of 140, I might've shoved the whole thing aside and forgotten about it. But according to Blood Sugar 101, those numbers were borderline. I was in the "pre-diabetic" range. Gradually I began restricting carbohydrates, frequently checking in with the glucose meter to ensure I was staying "in range". I would still eat plenty of carbohydrates, certainly not the 50g or 100g max that some seem to recommend. I wanted my food to be enjoyable. I figured I was genetically fortunate with a higher "carbohydrate tolerance".

My deterioration did not happen quickly. Sometimes we don't realize something is taking over our life if it happens slowly. Although I did not understand what was happening at the time, my restriction of carbohydrates was causing my glucose metabolism to down-regulate. Little by little that number on the glucose meter would inch upwards and I would reluctantly restrict a bit more.

Over the course of two years my diet and exercise patterns became completely obsessive. I learned that burning the glycogen stores in your muscles leads to a higher "carb tolerance" for several hours afterword. I learned that sugar does not cause as high a spike in the blood sugar. I got to a point where I was doing several hundred calories worth of cardio a day plus weight lifting two or three times a week. A number of disordered behaviors and red flags began to manifest. I would bring my own food with me when staying at my parents. I would get unduly worried if people decided to go to Dairy Queen. I was at my lowest weight ever and proud of my leanness, but my mother and girlfriend at the time had both commented independently that I looked "anorexic".

On top of the exercise I'd begun reading up on materials from the Weston A. Price Foundation. Not only did not my diet need to be low-carb, it needed to source high quality products from small farms. I was paying top dollar for a diet high in meat, butter, eggs, and sausage. Not only was the diet obsessive, it was expensive.

I didn't realize at first that the health problems I was experiencing were in any way related to diet. I've had insomnia off and on throughout my life, so when it started manifesting again, I basically cursed my luck and went on with things. The insomnia was proving to be a much bigger problem than it ever had been previously, and eventually, reluctantly, I started taking over the counter sleep medication. This helped for a while, but eventually I ended up talking to a sleep specialist and was prescribed Lunesta. I started this out sporadically at first, taking one every few days at most, but that soon increased as well.

It's hard to say how messed up I was by the end of everything. I would have two to four alcoholic drinks a night (a pattern I have never had before or since). My sleep was shot. On the worst days it felt like there was almost a "creepy crawly" or "raw nerve" type of sensation that would occur throughout my body. I began skipping out on activities. I wanted to turn in between eight and nine, solely for the hope I would get decent sleep and not feel horrible the next day.

During all of this I was continuing to dig deeper into health and nutrition. I'd contacted the University of Minnesota's School of Epidemiology about some questions I had about Ancel Keys' Seven Countries Study. A man there referred me to the book *The Cholesterol Wars* by Daniel Steinberg. Although expensive and scientifically dense, I needed to understand the mainstream arguments against fat and saturated fat in greater detail. Studying The Cholesterol Wars was not easy and I spent many months reading, thinking, taking notes, and looking up information online. I started to develop a much deeper understanding of LDL, cholesterol, and heart disease. The book, in my opinion, never proved its premise. The more I studied it, the more saturated fat appeared protective, and the more polyunsaturated fats seemed harmful. I began working on an extensive review of the book, which I was going to post on Amazon, when I suddenly stumbled across Chris Masterjohn's review. Chris's review already contained all the criticisms I was going to level at Steinberg, plus was already well researched and referenced. I stopped working on my review.

As much as I may have been learning, that period of research only served to reinforce my commitment to low-carb. It wasn't until I stumbled across Matt Stone's post on the Fathead blog I began seriously doubting the science behind it. Matt seemed to be directly contradicting things Taubes had "proven." I picked up some of his eBooks and began reading the wealth of contradictory evidence to all the low-carb dogma. I couldn't believe it. Had this evidence been lying around the whole time? How could Taubes and others so bullocksed it up as to not present any of this? How could I have been so daft as to essentially fall prey to the same illogical type of reasoning that was behind the anti-fat movement? Oh, the irony.

I remember the day I decided to quit low-carb and start Matt's "High Everything Diet" (HED). It was February 19th, 2010, at the Sustainable Farming Association of MN's annual conference. It was only two weeks after Matt's post on Fathead and we were being treated to the St. Olaf cafeteria, which features a large array of very tasty food. Over the next couple weeks my appetite became ravenous as my body sought to replace lean tissue mass. I would eat a generous portion of food for breakfast and then be starving three hours later. By the end of a month or so, I noticed I was growing a bit of a belly, and this started triggering all kinds of food inhibitions again.

One of my biggest concerns about restrictive diets now is the kind of mindset they put you in. You will have as much work undoing this mindset as you do healing your body. After a few months of less carbohydrate restriction, vastly reduced consumption of alcohol, caffeine, and sugar, and improved sleep, I was still having major problems with the "raw, crawly" type of skin sensations I described earlier. Between that and the fear of belly fat, I was not able to let go and achieve freedom around food. Instead, it's been a very long, very slow return to my old self, and I'm still not really there.

I spent two years slowly getting wrapped up in low-carb and becoming very orthorexic. I have now spent over two years trying to get back the way I was before I started. Things are far better now but only because I've continually learned to stop stressing over food and gradually incorporate the feedback my body's giving me. The strange symptoms I acquired from my low-carb stint were a big inhibition to my social life. Only recently, within the past couple months, have I felt well enough to stay out late or go to a party. Even here I am careful as a bad night's sleep or too much alcohol could have me feeling unpleasant and squirmy the next day.

I have always had insomnia, but it never used to bother me like this. If I wanted to go out with friends and they stayed up until four that was not a problem. I could still crash on a couch and feel decent the next day. What I developed during low-carb was of an altogether different character. I hesitate to even call it insomnia, which was probably only incidental. It is more likely I experienced underlying problems, such as nutrient depletion, disruption to hormonal or regulatory systems, or something similar. Having read through many former diet stories on Matt's blog, I realize now how long it can take these things to heal, and how much time and effort people spend trying to sort them out.

Anonymous

Just thought I'd drop you an email about my life on a paleo diet.

I'm now 35 and I've been working in the industry for 15 years. At first I hit upon set point theory after studying at Loughborough Uni and realising that as long as you pretty much stick to a pattern the body will regulate itself. So I did an experiment on myself and ate 6000 calories a day for a year. As you can imagine my metabolic rate went through the roof and the by-product of living my life on fast forward was that I started aging rapidly. I also lost a hell of a lot of weight and ended up at 10 stone.

At the time I was at the end of a career as a MTB rider, not the XC endurance style though. I did trials (on bikes and motorbikes) so was always pretty muscly from manhandling the bike around. At 10 stone I looked like I was dying, I actually did a few TV shows around that time with a few female pop groups who were always in the media being accused of eating disorders and they looked fat next to me.

So I was ripe for the paleo conversion, I knew how to manipulate weight loss but this seemed to offer the health I needed so badly. I have Asperger's so I'm pretty much a person that follows logic, which on the surface paleo seems to be. My Asperger's also means I love routine so I can honestly say that I lived the paleo lifestyle 100% of the time for around 8 years and I think that puts me in a good position to evaluate its performance.

I started out studying with CHEK, and I have nothing but praise for their teachings, both Paul and Dr Oliver taught me a hell of a lot about signs and symptoms of dysfunction. The problem came after studying, forums etc whipped up a storm with research backing the logic that we would or should all be "protein types". Over the years my belief led more and more problems with carbs. So I avoided anything other than my "allowed foods".

Initially the results were great, for a year I looked and felt amazing, but then you would if you'd previously been 10 stone. The results slowly faded and I never looked that good again. I still "thought" I felt good though despite the worrying signs I had developed xanthelasma in the corner of my eyes, loss of outer 1/3rd of my eyebrow and lower shin hair. I ignored this because I was focused on the "pot belly", and to cut a long story short I became more and more extreme chasing those initial results. The only times I saw better results were during my trips to America where I could get organic berries and organic green apples (the ones allowed when I did MT and not available in the UK). Whenever I came to the states I'd lose the pot belly but could never figure out why. I put it down to finally getting some carbs and to increased variety.

Last year it was all coming to a head, my own wedding had made me look weird because I needed my own meal cooking to accommodate my strange diet. I had various aches and pains, still had my pot belly and my wife was concerned about my raised cholesterol levels. I began studying for an MSc in Psychology in particular looking at health/food.

Then out of the blue my right achilles fully ruptured, followed shortly later by a blood clot, pulmonary embolism and a lung infarction that should of killed me. When I came round in the resuscitation room of the ER my first thoughts were that I was "healthy" and that it shouldn't be happening to me. In the hospital the books came out and by the end of the first week in the hospital I was once again eating sugar. Upon leaving the hospital I had a consultation with an RBTI practitioner who told me my connective tissue was brittle and that I had thick blood. This was enough to kick some sense into me and allow me to realise that my dalliance with paleo/MT was more than likely a psychological condition or an eating disorder. I firmly believed that I scared myself almost to death worrying about foods for absolutely no benefit.

Anonymous

My nutrition story is a long one with plenty of diet fails along the way.

I was a normal kid growing up, eating what normal kids ate. Plenty of healthy foods and plenty of junk as well. I was always active and stayed lean up until around 19. That's when I stopped doing sports and took up drinking and video games. From 19 until 22 I did little else besides drink, play games and eat garbage. I went from a lean 170 to a real chubby 215. The worst part was I had never lifted weights before that so it was all fat. One day I remember someone told me that a girl I knew was talking about how fat I had gotten, that hit me hard and kicked me in the ass to do something, and I did. I started starving myself while doing miles and miles on the treadmill. I also lifted weights daily and within a couple of months I dropped right back down to about 180 with no real problems whatsoever. I felt great and looked good. I almost had abs! This was the beginning of the shit storm of misinformation that is the health and nutrition world.

I decided to take things further and started reading all sorts of blogs and websites aimed at fitness and nutrition. I don't remember how I came across MarksDailyApple but I do remember that I thought I had opened the holy grail. Everything I read made so much sense. Sugar drives insulin drives fat. So simple! Grains were actually the devil! It didn't matter that I had eaten them my entire life. The science was there and that was that. I immediately went full bore. I bought

Cordains book, read Marks website and a few others and was hooked. For the next 8 months my diet consisted of plenty of meat and eggs, boat loads of veggies and handfuls of nuts every couple of hours. Once in a while I would throw in some fruit but only after I did some Crossfit type workout!

Well like everyone's paleo story, I felt great! Sure I had some tiredness and some really bad soreness that didn't seem to want to go away, but that was probably just detoxing from the crap I had eaten my whole life.

Around the ninth month mark I started feeling pretty bad. My libido dropped to pretty much nothing. My feet, and lower back among other things started getting very painful. It was impossible for me to recover from working out and I couldn't even run because my joints didn't want to work right. Well I didn't understand it and by this time I was deeply entrenched in the paleo dogma. I decided I wasn't being strict enough so I started eliminating other things and narrowed my diet down to meat and veggies. I also threw in some fasting for good measure. Things kept getting worse... Finally I found what I thought was the answer to my problems when I stumbled across a thread posting by a man named "Bear" who had been eating nothing but meat for years and was thriving! So I tried it.

9 days on an all meat diet when everything went terribly wrong. I started getting severe abdominal pains, I couldn't lay down because the bed made my joints too sore to sleep. I didn't know what to do so I went to the doctor. Nothing. I went home, pretty depressed. By the way, this was about 3-4 years into my paleo madness. Ihad actually put on about 20lbs since the beginning even though I was eating at a deficit. The very same day that I went to the doctor, I remembered reading about someone by the name of Matt Stone who was talking shit to one of my favorite bloggers by the name of Richard. When I

first read it I just shrugged him off as a wack job but for some reason I remembered him talking about the paleo diet being a bad idea so I googled him, found his site and read his entire ebook that night. The next day I put it into practice. Started eating everything I had been missing out on for years and then some.

A few things happened that first week that really made me pause. One… my abdominal pain went away. My joint pains also went down by quite a bit but the thing that really threw me for a loop was that my man boobs almost went away completely. This proved to me that there were some hormonal issues going on. This isn't the end of my story though because a couple weeks into stuffing my face, my abdominal pain came back. Same pain I had had on an all meat diet. I was perplexed and disappointed. I did not know what could be causing it. By this time I was reading up on websites that were on the other end of the spectrum like Ray Peat and 30bananasaday.com. Then one night it clicked, the thing that RRARF and an all meat diet have in common is the meat and fat! The very thing I held as the standard of a healthy diet was the thing nearly putting me in the hospital. Meat and fat.

The next day I ate nothing but fruit. I felt amazing. The next 4 days I ate nothing but fruit. Amazing. Then I got sick of fruit. I think it was about this time that I wrote to Matt and got some advice. I decided I would try something I haven't thought of doing in over 5 years. I would eat a high carb, low fat/low protein diet. I mixed in a lot of Peat's ideas and my diet ended up consisting mostly of grains, dairy and fruit. Recently it has expanded to meat and eggs a couple times a week but I don't exclude anything entirely, just try to keep PUFA, veggies, meat and other fats at a minimum.

Well the rest is history. This was close to a year ago I believe and I finally know I found out what works for me. I no longer have joint pain or inflammation of any kind, no longer suffer from lack of energy or low libido. I usually get in one weight training session a day, sometimes two and I recover from them within the day. I sleep like a baby without waking up once. On the paleo diet I was getting up 3-5 times a night to pee. I am still a work in progress. I don't have a six pack yet but I am sitting at around 200lbs with a ton more muscle than I have ever had in my life. When I do dial everything in I will be sure to share my progress.

Scott from Bro-Cal

Here is my paleo story, do with it what you will.
A bit of background: 21 year old college student in southern California, became interested in health and nutrition when I started developing eczema after raging in the frat castle for over 3 years. Good Bowel movements, above average body temperature (usually very warm at night had all windows open and ceiling fan on full blast) and tons of energy for "raging my face off."

It started off as a near ordinary day, when my eczema was breaking out once again. (At this point this was my only problem to speak of, the fairytale goes south soon my children). I found a website that discussed treatment methods and one of them said a lowish carb diet with plenty of homemade kefir and coconut oil. At first I was skeptical, how can food effect our lives that substantially? Can this anti-candida diet really do the trick? I must have candida it is the only explanation! The first couple days were whatever but then by day 4 I was peeing out my butt (pardon my french) and the eczema was changing from less of a rash to something much redder. Like most people I kept reading about die off and all the awesome stuff that happens because of it. Frequent urination, anxiety started to build up, overall mood went down. I figured this is what I was going through, but still the probiotics were giving me the worst gas of my life so I lowered the dose (people keep promoting this stuff to everybody as a panacea to all your problems, all it gave me was bad gas and heart burn).

But wait how does this relate to paleo? Well About 2 months later I gave up and started eating rice and fruit again along with eating out and only ordering french fries. Things were getting a lot better, no more coldness in hands, less muscle pain, etc. Here's the turning point my children, I discovered the crown jewel of health, marks daily apple. It was beautiful when I first found this lost city in the heart of the amazon. In the golden treasure chest was a manuscript that simply said, "Remove grains, Dairy, and legumes from diet and obey the 80/20 rule, this my son is the true meaning of life and happiness."

Of Course it all seems so simple now, the advent of agriculture was killing us all, who cares if my hair is thinning and my skin is becoming progressively drier? So I tossed the grains and french fries and I went full on rocking out with my Grok out.

The Grok Wars Part 1: A New Diet

I think I was spending close to $100 a week at whole foods on vegetables alone, nothing could satisfy and potatoes are bad we all know that. The cognitive abilities began to fail in my brain pretty quick. Easy college classes quickly became eye sores, the thought of talking with those less fortunate of not hearing the message of the primal wisdom made me irritated about how much they didn't know about the government's plan to destroy us all (at this point I felt like I was on LSD half the time, hippie living the 70's life of lots of vegetables and conspiracy theories). I barely made it through that semester. I was going #2 twice in one morning, light-headed, shortness of breath, still urinating more than usual but hey I was ripped, not an ounce of body fat. However this came with a cost. I started lifting heavy things without enough carbohydrates, bad move sparky. Developed a tingling sensation in my back that spread to my arms, legs and neck. At this point I was concerned for the first time, although I should have been before after spending 4 months in near ketosis. I started going to see doctors, naturopaths, etc explaining my candida story and how grok was the answer to all my problems. All they saw was malnourished white kid who had too much on his plate and too many ideas about health and nutrition that were driving him insane. Weight at that point was 130 (normal would be 150). The semester ended and I decided it was time to head home to Big Steve's (my dad) house and figure out wtf was going on.

The Grok Wars Part 2: The Diet Strikes Back

Endless nights spent on the computer looking for answers became the norm, no bar hopping or hooking up with random chicks anymore. I stumbled across more primal wisdom, started ordering a bunch of books, but no matter what I read I just had this biased opinion about carbs. Bad logic from books like Paul Chek's *Eat, Move, and Be Healthy* along with paleo favorites like *The Vegetarian Myth* and *Primal Body, Primal Mind* further solidified my findings that grok was the way to go.

I ended up in the emergency room when my head started to spin and my heart rate was through the roof. I went to more doctors and they told me that I have high cholesterol and that I should consider going on a diet (I thought I was on one?). The medical bills were piling up and the pain in my back, stomach, and head would just not quit. Memory loss and inability to recall past events left me mentally crippled as reading words or memorizing song lyrics would just not register in the memory banks. Then midway through the summer, I broke down hard and with whatever mental clarity I had left, something spoke to me and said hey "dumbass, remember when we used to eat taco bell and a big fat bowl of spaghetti?" I responded to my inner thoughts, "yea I remember those days, they were awesome." It was at that moment that I went back to 180 Degree Health after first dismissing it and read through a couple articles. I said "F^&K It" and the healing chapter began.

The Grok Wars Part 3: The Return of the Taco Bell

It was time. I picked up my light saber and went back to master yoda's planet realizing that my training was not complete regarding nutrition and overall well-being. The first couple days of normal eating felt like I was in Las Vegas snorting cocaine. My Feet and face were on fire, I had so much energy again it was literally stupid but the crashes from all the pizza and Gatorade were redonkulous. It felt like kindergarten all over again, Nap time was alllllllllll the time. However my relationship with food continued to grow stronger. Taco bell and myself were BFF's again and I even hooked up with an ex-food lover of my mine on a daily basis, yup me and spaghetti and meatballs had it made. The pressure in my head was lessening and mental abilities started to come back. I was known amongst my friends as the stat man. I could memorize baseball stats so easily and remember them years later.

My Jedi powers started to return to me as I argued baseball at the bars until the wee hours of the morning like a true Jedi Warrior. Alcohol was hard to bring back at first as at this point I could have half a beer and have a pretty good buzz going, to the point where I would throw things and scream profanities at strangers....talk about a 1 beer queer. 6 months down the road and while I would say I'm feeling better but I am nowhere near the frat star I was before. I have a feeling it will take some time for me to regain my powers, but I have destroyed the evil empire in my thought process and the death star is no longer lingering over my head. Although the Dark side of the Grok will tempt others and it will feed off of their desperation and anger just like it did to me, there is always hope that those individuals will come back to the light side of the force or what most of us call planet earth and not the grokosphere.

Overall this experience has been one giant boner kill, but I have gained knowledge from this experience that I would not have found otherwise. Maybe I will look back at this in future and laugh but for now I'm still feeling the after burn.

Other Books and Audio Programs by Matt Stone

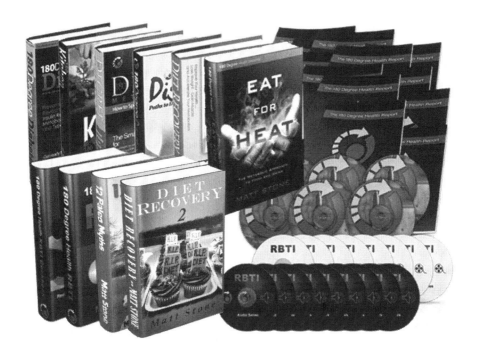

Save $9.99 towards the purchase of the 180 Platinum Collection, a collection of the principal 180DegreeHealth materials by…

- Going online to: http://180degreehealth.com/180-degree-health-store
- Clicking on "The 180 Platinum Collection"
- Adding it to your cart
- Entering the discount code "abab"
- Pressing the "Update Cart" Button
- And proceeding through checkout

References

The assertions made in *12 Paleo Myths* are a comprehensive culmination of conclusions pieced together, in part, by a thorough and critical examination of the following books, websites, and articles (although this is most certainly just a partial list):

Abrahamson, E. M. and A. W. Pezet. *Body, Mind, and Sugar.* Avon Books: New York, NY, 1951.

Agatston, Arthur. *The South Beach Diet.* Rodale: New York, NY, 2003.

Allan, Christian B. and Wolfgang Lutz. *Life Without Bread.* Keats Publishing: Los Angeles, CA, 2000.

Appleton, Nancy. *Stopping Inflammation.* Square One Publishers: Garden City Park, NY, 2005.

Appleton, Nancy. *Suicide By Sugar.* Square One Publishers: Garden City Park, NY, 2009.

Atkins, Robert. *Dr. Robert Atkins New Diet Revolution.* Avon Books, Inc.: New York, NY, 1992.

Aziz, Michael. *The Perfect 10 Diet.* Cumberland House: Naperville, IL, 2010.

Bacon, Linda. *Health at Every Size.* Benbella Books: Dallas, TX, 2008.

Barnard, Neal. *Dr. Neal Barnard's Program for Reversing Diabetes.* Rodale: New

York, NY, 2007.

Barnes, Broda. *Hypothyroidism: The Unsuspecting Illness.* Harper and Row: New York, NY, 1976

Barnes, Broda. *Solved: The Riddle of Heart Attacks.* Robinson Press: Fort Collins, CO, 1976

Barnes, Broda. *Hope for Hypoglycemia.* Robinson Press: Fort Collins, CO, 1978

Bass, Clarence. *Great Expectations.* Ripped Enterprises: Albuquerque, NM, 2007.

Bennett, Connie. *Sugar Shock!* Berkley Books: New York, NY, 2007.

Bieler, Henry. *Food is Your Best Medicine.* Random House: New York, NY, 1965.

Brownstein, David. *Overcoming Thyroid Disorders.* Medical Alternative Press: West Bloomfield, MI, 2008.

Burkitt, Denis, Hugh Trowell, and Kenneth Heaton. *Dietary Fibre, Fibre-Depleted Foods and Disease.* Academic Press: London, 1985.

Campos, Paul. *The Obesity Myth.* Gotham Books: New York, NY, 2004.

Challem, Jack. *The Inflammation Syndrome.* John Wiley and Sons, Inc.: Hoboken, NJ, 2003.

Chilton, Floyd H. *Inflammation Nation.* Fireside: New York, NY, 2007.

Cleave, T. L., *The Saccharine Disease*. Keats Publishing: New Canaan, CT, 1974.

Cleave, T.L. and G.D. Campbell. *Diabetes, Coronary Thrombosis, and the Saccharine Disease*. John Wright & Sons LTD.: Bristol, UK, 1969.

Cochran, Gregory and Henry Harpending. *The 10,000 Year Explosion*. Basic Books: New York, NY, 2009.

Colpo, Anthony. *The Fat Loss Bible*.

Cordain, Loren. *The Paleo Diet*. John Wiley & Sons: Hoboken, NJ, 2002.

Cordain, Loren and Joe Friel. *The Paleo Diet for Athletes*. Rodale: New York, NY, 2005.

DesMaisons, Kathleen. *Potatoes Not Prozac*. Fireside: New York, NY, 1998.

DesMaisons, Kathleen. *The Sugar Addict's Total Recovery Program*. Ballantine Books: New York, NY, 2000.

De Vany, Arthur. *The New Evolution Diet*. Rodale: New York, NY, 2011.

Dufty, William. *Sugar Blues*. Warner Books: New York, NY, 1975.

Eades, Michael R. and Mary Dan. *Protein Power*. Bantam Books: New York, NY, 1996.

Ellis, Gregory. *Dr. Ellis's Ultimate Diet Secrets Lite*. Targeted Body Systems Publishing: Glen Mills, PA, 2003.

Enig, Mary. *Know Your Fats.* Bethesda Press: Silver Spring, MD, 2000.

Farris, Russell and Per Marin. *The Potbelly Syndrome.* Basic Health Publications:
Laguna Beach, CA, 2006.

Fife, Bruce. *Eat Fat Look Thin.* Healthwise: Colorado Springs, CO, 2002.

Fife, Bruce. *The Coconut Oil Miracle.* Avery: New York, NY, 1999.

Fraser, Laura. *Losing It.* Plume: New York, NY, 1997.

Fuhrman, Joel. *Eat to Live.* Little, Brown and Company: New York, NY, 2003.

Gabriel, Jon. *The Gabriel Method.* Atria Books: New York, NY, 2008.

Galland, Leo. *The Fat Resistance Diet.* Broadway Books: New York, NY, 2005.

Gedgaudas, Nora. *Primal Body, Primal Mind.* Primal Body – Primal Mind Publishing: Portland, OR, 2009.

Johnson, Richard J. *The Sugar Fix.* Pocket Books: New York, NY, 2008.

Keys, Ancel et al. *The Biology of Human Starvation.* The University of Minnesota Press: Minneapolis, MN, 1950.

Kharrazian, Datis. *Why Do I Still Have Thyroid Symptoms?* Morgan James Publishing: Garden City, NY, 2010.

Kolata, Gina. *Rethinking Thin.* Farrar, Straus and Giroux: New York, NY, 2007.

Langer, Stpehen E. and James F. Scheer. *Solved: The Riddle of Illness.* McGraw Hill: New York, NY, 2006.

Lindeberg, Staffan. *Food and Western Disease.* Wiley-Blackwell: West Sussex, UK, 2010.

Lipton, Bruce. *The Biology of Belief.* Elite Books: Santa Rosa, CA, 2005.

Macfadden, Bernarr. *The Miracle of Milk.* Macfadden Publications: New York, NY, 1924.

Martin, Courtney E. *Perfect Girls, Starving Daughters.* Free Press: New York, NY, 2007.

McCarrison, Robert. *Studies in Deficiency Disease.* Henry Frowde and Hodder and Stoughton: London, England, 1921.

McCully, Kilmer S. *The Homocysteine Revolution.* Keats Publishing: New Canaan, CT, 1997.

McDonald, Lyle. *Ultimate Diet 2.0*

Morris, Richard. *A Life Unburdened.* New Trends Publishing: Washington, D.C., 2007.

Murray, Michael. *The Encyclopedia of Healing Foods.* Atria Books: New York, NY, 2005.

Paula Owens. *The Power of 4.* Paula Owens: USA. 2008.

Page, Melvin, and H. Leon Abrams. *Health vs. Disease*, The Page Foundation, Inc., St. Petersburg, FL 1960.

Peat, Ray. *Progesterone in Orthomolecular Medicine.* Raymond Peat: Eugene, OR, 1993.

Peat, Ray. *Generative Energy.* Raymond Peat: Eugene, OR, 1994.

Peat, Ray. *Nutrition for Women.* Raymond Peat: Eugene, OR, 1993.

Peat, Ray. *Mind and Tissue.* Raymond Peat: Eugene, OR, 1993.

Peat, Ray. *From PMS to Menopause.* Raymond Peat: Eugene, OR, 1993.

Pekarek, Martha L. *Freedom from Obesity and Sugar Addiction.* Wheatmark: Tucson, AZ, 2007.

Philpott, William H. *Victory Over Diabetes.* Keats Publishing: New Canaan, CT, 1983.

Pool, Robert. *Fat: Fighting the Obesity Epidemic.* Oxford University Press: New York, NY, 2001.

Porter, Charles Sanford. *Milk Diet, as a Remedy for Chronic Disease.* Burnett P.O.: Long Beach, CA, 1916.

Price, Weston A. *Nutrition and Physical Degeneration.* Republished by the Price-
Pottenger Nutrition Foundation: La Mesa, CA, originally published in 1939.

Reaven, Gerald. *Syndrome X.* Fireside: New York, NY, 2000.

Roberts, Seth. *The Shangri-La Diet.* G. P. Putnam's Sons: New York, NY, 2006.

Rooney, Ric. *Secrets of a Professional Dieter* (eBook). www.PhysiqueTransformation.com

Ross, Julia. *The Diet Cure.* Penguin Books: New York, NY, 1999.

Shell, Ellen Ruppel. *The Hungry Gene.* Atlantic Monthly Press: New York, NY, 2002.

Schmid, Ron. *Traditional Foods are Your Best Medicine.* Healing Arts Press:
Rochester, VT, 1987.

Schwartz, Bob. *Diets Don't Work!* Breakthrough Publishing: Houston, TX, 1982.

Schwarzbein, Diana. *The Schwarzbein Principle.* Health Communications, Inc.:
Deerfield Beach, FL, 1999.

Schwarzbein, Diana. *The Schwarzbein Principle II.* Health Communications, Inc.: Deerfield Beach, FL, 2002.

Schwarzbein, Diana. *The Program.* Health Communications, Inc.: Deerfield Beach, FL, 2004.

Selye, Hans. *The Stress of Life.* McGraw-Hill: New York, NY, 1976.

Sears, Al. *P.A.C.E.* Wellness Research and Consulting, Inc.: Royal Palm Beach, FL, 2010.

Sears, Barry. *Enter the Zone.* Regan Books: New York, NY, 1995.

Sears, Barry. *The Age-Free Zone.* Regan Books: New York, NY, 1999.

Sears, Barry. *The Anti-Inflammation Zone.* Collins: New York, NY, 2005.

Sears, Barry. *Toxic Fat.* Thomas Nelson Inc, 2008.

Shell, Ellen Ruppel. *The Hungry Gene.* Atlantic Monthly Press: New York, NY, 2002.

Shomon, Mary J., *The Thyroid Diet.* Harper Resource: New York, NY, 2004.

Sisson, Mark. *The Primal Blueprint.* Primal Nutrition, Inc.: Malibu, CA, 2009.

Starr, Mark. *Hypothyroidism Type II.* Mark Starr Trust: Columbia, MO, 2005.

Talbott, Shawn. *The Cortisol Connection.* Hunter House: Alameda, CA, 2007.

Taubes, Gary. *Good Calories, Bad Calories.* Alfred A. Knopf: New York, NY, 2007.

Tribole, Evelyn and Elyse Resch. *Intuitive Eating.* St. Martin's Press: New York, NY, 1995.

Wann, Marilyn. *Fat?So!* Ten Speed Press: Berkeley, CA, 1998.

Weil, Andrew. *Eating Well for Optimum Health.* Harper Collins: New York, NY, 2000.

Wiley, T.S. *Lights Out: Sleep, Sugar, and Survival.* Pocket Books: New York, NY,

2000.

Wolf, Robb. *The Paleo Solution.* Victory Belt: Las Vegas, NV, 2010.

Wrangham, Richard. *Catching Fire.* Basic Books: New York, NY, 2009.

Yudkin, John. *Sweet and Dangerous.* Bantam Books: New York, NY, 1972.

Websites:
www.raypeat.com
http://nutritionscienceanalyst.blogspot.com/
www.stopthethyroidmadness.com
http://thescientificdebateforum.aimoo.com/
www.wholehealthsource.blogspot.com
www.omega-6-news.org
http://blog.cholesterol-and-health.com/
www.westonaprice.org
www.carbsanity.blogspot.com
www.weightology.net
www.sethroberts.net
www.junkfoodscience.blogspot.com
www.scottabel.com
www.leangains.com
www.30bananasaday.com
www.youtube.com/durianriders

A Few Specific Article and video titles with accompanying URLs:

"Depressive Symptoms, omega-6:omega-3 Fatty Acids, and Inflammation in Older Adults"

http://www.psychosomaticmedicine.org/cgi/content/abstract/69/3/217

"Suppressor of Cytokine Signaling-3 (SOCS-3), a Potential Mediator of Interleukin-6-dependent Insulin Resistance in Hepatocytes"

http://www.jbc.org/content/278/16/13740.full.pdf

"Eluv Live Interview with Dr. Ray Peat"
http://eluv.podbean.com/2008/10/10/eluv-live-interview-with-dr-ray-peat/
"Obesity: 10 Things You Thought You Knew"
http://www.youtube.com/watch?v=Qk4UKD00aOo&feature=channel
"The Ghost in Your Genes"
http://video.google.com/videoplay?docid=1128045835761675934#

Suggested Reading
180 Degree Metabolism by Matt Stone
Health at Every Size by Linda Bacon
The Obesity Myth by Paul Campos
Hypothyroidism: The Unsuspecting Illness by Broda Barnes
The Cortisol Connection by Shawn Talbott
Hypothyroidism Type 2: The Epidemic by Mark Starr
http://wholehealthsource.blogspot.com
www.raypeat.com

About the Author

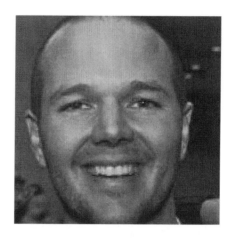

Matt Stone is the founder of 180DegreeHealth. He is an independent health researcher and author of more than 10 books, including multiple titles that have made it to #1 in their respective categories on Amazon. Most of his research has drawn him towards metabolic rate and how many basic functions (digestion, reproduction, aging, immunity, inflammation, mood, circulation, sleep) perform better when metabolic rate is optimized. He is most notable for his criticisms of extreme diets and exposing many false diet industry claims, as well as his works on raising metabolic rate through simple changes in diet and lifestyle. His views and findings are discussed exhaustively on the site and cataloged in many of Stone's books available for sale through Amazon.